Vision Impairment

Vision Impairment

Science, art and lived experience

Michael Crossland

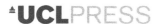

First published in 2024 by
UCL Press
University College London
Gower Street
London WC1E 6BT

Available to download free: www.uclpress.co.uk

A CIP catalogue record for this book is available from The British Library.

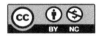

ISBN: 978-1-80008-624-1 (Hbk.)
ISBN: 978-1-80008-623-4 (Pbk.)
ISBN: 978-1-80008-622-7 (PDF)
ISBN: 978-1-80008-625-8 (epub)
DOI: https://doi.org/10.14324/111.9781800086227

To Kate and Simone, with love

Contents

List of figures

List of tables

Preface

Since training as an optometrist in the 1990s, I have worked with thousands of people with severe vision impairment and I am often asked 'what is it *really* like to go blind?' This book is my attempt to answer this huge question, using research from low vision laboratories across the globe, art made by people with vision loss, depictions of blind people in literature, and my experiences from working in the low vision clinic of one of the world's leading eye hospitals, in London.

In the hospital, I divide my time between children's and adults' low vision clinics. The people I meet in the clinic have significant vision loss, ranging from those whose vision is just too poor to legally drive a car, to those who can barely see a very bright light. I use various techniques to improve their visual function, such as prescribing high-power spectacles, providing magnifiers and telescopes, advising on technology, and referring them to counsellors, mobility instructors, rehabilitation workers and specialist teachers.

I am also a senior research fellow at UCL, where I work more deeply with people with vision impairment, investigating better ways to measure sight loss, evaluating new technology to help people with low vision and exploring the impact of vision impairment on wellbeing and mental health.

I have spent my working life around people with vision impairment, but I am not visually impaired. This puts me in a slightly awkward position, as in many ways the stories in this book are not mine to tell. I don't want this book to feel voyeuristic, nor do I want to exploit the experiences of people I have met in clinic. The academic Tom Shakespeare called Oliver Sacks 'the man who mistook his patients for a literary career' and this is certainly not my intention in writing this book. Instead, I am using these stories to explain what life is like for people with vision impairment and to present research in ophthalmology and low vision to a wider audience.

In Chapter 1, I discuss the word 'blindness', an emotive term that some people with vision impairment prefer not to use. After consideration, I have decided to include it in this book, as it is a word I hear so often in the clinic. I apologise for any discomfort created by my use of the 'b-word'. This chapter also explores the tricky question of how little vision someone needs to have to be described as blind and describes the major causes of sight loss throughout the world.

Chapter 2 looks at art created by people with vision impairment and ways in which artists, authors and poets have communicated their own sight loss. When I meet people who have been recently diagnosed with a blinding eye condition, their impression of what a blind person looks like very often comes from depictions on screen, usually by a sighted actor who is working from a set of cultural stereotypes. I examine some of the tropes associated with blindness and how they are portrayed in film, television, music and literature.

In the children's clinic, I am often asked which careers young people with vision impairment are able to follow. In Chapter 3, I describe many jobs that are successfully performed by people with significant sight loss, and look at the history of education and training for people with vision impairment.

Along with 'what is it like to go blind?', 'do blind people have better hearing?' is another frequently asked question. Chapter 4 looks at the interaction between vision impairment and performance on other senses and shows that, yes, in some circumstances, blind people do use their hearing more effectively. I describe how the brain adjusts when the input from one sense is reduced, reviewing recent advances in our understanding of the brain's visual system.

Chapter 5 continues looking at the role of the brain in vision and describes the (sometimes unusual) effects of brain disease on visual perception. This chapter also describes how the brain can create false images and hallucinations in some people with sight loss.

In Chapter 6, I look at the psychological impact of vision impairment, including the grieving process that people sometimes experience after losing their vision. Chapter 7 looks at some of the activities that people might pursue once they have adjusted to their sight loss, such as travelling and dating.

Finally, Chapter 8 explores some of the emerging treatments and therapies for some causes of vision impairment and asks whether artificial intelligence, gene therapy or even Google will mean that there will be fewer people with vision impairment in the future. The chapter closes by outlining the social and medical model of disability and asks what we would lose in a world without blind people.

The characters in this book are portmanteaus of many people I have met in the clinic, at conferences or as friends. Identifying details have been changed throughout, and this book should be read as a work of creative non-fiction. However, everyone named with their surname is a real person, and I have represented these people as accurately as I can.

Acknowledgements

When I was an undergraduate, I didn't realise I would specialise in vision impairment and only did so thanks to the inspirational guidance of some phenomenal clinicians and scientists. In approximately chronological order, these were: Keziah Latham, Louise Culham, Andrew Milliken, Janet Silver, Liz Gould, Catherine Grigg, Marek Karas, Michael Banes, Gary Rubin, Antonio Filipe Macedo, Dan Ehrlich, Mitch Reuben and Hannah Dunbar.

Thank you to Paul Laffan and Julie Garton from the writing department at City Lit and to the many friends who have read or heard early drafts of this book and kept me motivated, especially Kelly Carver, Patrick Griffiths, Gordon Legge, Nadeem Ali, Amber Butchart, Andy Curtis, Pete Finn, Jane Hutcheon, Darren Lee, Andrew Macalpine, Pam Schickler, Matt Shipton, Louise Skowron, Stephen Vaudrey and Ian Wishart. Chris Penfold at UCL Press has been an encouraging and supportive presence throughout this long project. It has been a pleasure to have my writing improved by such an engaged, professional and diligent editor.

While writing this book, I read dozens of memoirs and first-person stories about blindness. The one I would recommend above all others is *Sight Unseen* by Georgina Kleege. I was shocked that my university shelves this under 'art' rather than 'medicine', as it should be compulsory reading for everyone working with vision impaired people.

Thank you to Lenka Clayton, Luka Kille, Kelly and Lucia Carver and Jenni Turner for permission to include their artwork or writing in this book, and to Luka for being so generous with her time for interviews.

I would like to acknowledge the organisations which have supported my research work: Guide Dogs, the National Institute for Health Research, Innovate UK, Moorfields Eye Charity and the Macular Society. I am also grateful to Tessa Dekker and my colleagues in the UCL Child Vision Lab for their patience while my attention was with this manuscript!

Finally, I owe a debt of gratitude to everyone I meet in the low vision clinic. Whether or not I have included your story in this book, I have learnt something from each of you.

1
What is blindness?

'So would you say I'm blind?' Sam asked.

This sounds like a straightforward question. Sam had been attending my low vision clinic for six years, so surely I would be able to answer her without a second thought?

Sam had an eye condition called Stargardt disease, which was slowly causing the cells in the central part of her retina to stop working. Just after starting high school when she was 11, she had found it difficult to see the whiteboard in some of her classrooms. Assuming she needed an eye test, her parents took her to a local optometrist who prescribed spectacles, but they didn't seem to make much difference to her sight. Her family realised there was something seriously wrong when Sam asked for the ketchup bottle to be passed, not seeing that it was right in front of her. A trip to her doctor led to a referral to an eye hospital, blood tests, scans, photographs and the unwelcome news that she had a serious, inherited and generally untreatable eye disease.

Sam remembers the news being broken: 'The consultant just said "there's not a lot we can do",' she told me. 'I felt a bit like he was washing his hands of me, although I'm really pleased he referred me to this place.' 'This place' was the low vision clinic we were sitting in, buried away at the back of the hospital. At her previous visits to the clinic I had prescribed Sam strong reading spectacles, given her various magnifying glasses and shown her how to set up her iPhone to make it easier to see. I'd spoken to her specialist teacher for visual impairment to make sure she had a relay system for the whiteboard at school, and had given her details for a group so she could meet other teenagers with sight loss. Since her first visit, Sam had changed from being a shy and slightly awkward girl to a rebellious teenager (an appearance not helped by the way that her vision loss made it difficult to maintain eye contact), then a funny and engaging young adult. Now she had green hair and wore Doc Martens, a denim jacket and a 'Meat is Murder' T-shirt.

Sam's question about whether I would call her 'blind' may have been spurred on by the fact that her vision had clearly got worse. For the first time, she could no longer make out the letters on the top row of my sight chart, four metres away from her. When I wheeled the chart closer to Sam she could read the first few letters by moving her eyes around, sliding the blind area in the central part of her vision away from what she was looking at and using her peripheral retina to just about see.

Sam had told me that she'd got the grades she wanted in her A Levels and that she was very excited about moving to Leeds to study politics. She'd told me that her football team had won a tournament that summer and that she'd started a band with some of her college friends. She could travel independently, using apps on her phone to help when she couldn't see a bus number or platform sign. Her vision was too poor to have a driving licence, but she could cycle to band rehearsals. She'd had enlarged print and additional time in her exams, but she didn't read braille or have a guide dog. Would this active and successful teenager meet most people's idea of a blind person? The poet Stephen Kuusisto talks about people entering 'the planet of the blind',[1] but would Sam be welcome there?

The word 'blind' is emotionally charged and tends to be avoided by people working in eye clinics. In the UK, being 'registered blind' was replaced in the early 2000s with 'having a certificate of vision impairment'. In ophthalmology research, we even speak about 'double masked trials' rather than the 'double blind' studies used in other areas of medicine.

This coyness around the word 'blind' isn't universal. Many of the major sight loss charities use the word in their names, such as the UK's Royal National Institute of Blind People, the National Association for the Blind in India and New Zealand's Blind and Low Vision NZ. In 2011, the London-based Metropolitan Society for the Blind renamed themselves 'Blind Aid', which almost feels like reclaiming the word for people with vision impairment.

Writer Georgina Kleege uses the word 'blind' as she dislikes the alternatives: 'The word "impairment" implies impermanence ... but my condition has no cure or treatment ... I crave the simplicity of a single, unmodified adjective. Blind. Perhaps I could speak in relative terms, say I am blinder than some, less blind than others.'[2] Kleege has only come to embrace the word 'blind' after several decades of low vision. She writes that as a teenager 'the most I would admit to was a "problem with my eyes", sometimes adding, "and they won't give me glasses", indicating that it was not me but the wilfully obstructionist medical establishment which was to blame for my failure to see as I should'.

When Sam asked if she was blind, I heard her father gently whistle at the gravity of the question. The room was so small that I thought I could feel his breath on the back of my neck. The background hum of the busy clinic around me seemed to drop, as if everyone was waiting for my response. Even as I spoke, I knew my answer was a cop out:

'The word "blind" means something different to nearly everyone I meet,' I told her. 'We prefer to say "severely sight impaired". It's true that if you were in America you'd be called "legally blind", but you're certainly someone who uses your eyes for most things, so I don't think "blind" would be the best word to describe you.'

'Legally blind,' Sam said, almost under her breath. I thought she was going to comment on this dramatic label, but she surprised me instead. 'We've been looking for a name for our band, and I think that might be it!'

How blind is blind?

Most people probably would not see Sam and think 'There goes a blind woman,' which raises the question: how well can someone see but still be classified as 'blind'? Would anyone whose vision is too poor to drive qualify as blind? What about someone with advanced tunnel vision, who can see small details but only in one tiny pinpoint of the world? What if someone is so sensitive to light that they can't leave the house in the daytime, even when wearing the darkest sunglasses? Or should the word 'blind' be reserved for people who don't see any light at all, who can't say whether a room light is switched on or off?

When I think about how well someone sees, I think about two factors: the smallest size of object they can see (their visual acuity) and how far they can see around them (their visual field).

Visual acuity

Visual acuity is usually measured with a Snellen chart: the common test seen in high street opticians' practices, doctor's surgeries and eye clinics – so familiar that it's even used as a shorthand for an eye examination in cartoons. The largest letter at the top of the chart is

10 times bigger than the standard of 'good vision', so somebody who can only see the top letter has a visual acuity about 10 times poorer than someone without eye disease. The letters towards the bottom of the chart are given the size '6', which means they can be read by someone with good sight from six metres. Someone reading these letters has a visual acuity of 6/6 in the UK, or 20/20 in the USA, where their dislike of the metric system means the chart is placed at 20 feet rather than six metres. Another person who can only see the top letter has a visual acuity of 6/60, or 20/200, meaning they can see from six metres objects of the same size that we would expect to be seen from 60 metres. Put another way, things need to be 10 times larger, or they need to be 10 times closer, for them to see them as well as someone with good sight.

Since the Snellen chart was invented in 1862 it has been used all over the world, with versions using pictures, numbers, Cyrillic, Japanese and Arabic print. The image below (Figure 1.1) shows a sight chart being used outside an eye clinic in Tanzania, with a 'tumbling E' being used for people who are unable to read: the person taking the test indicates the direction of each letter E by holding their hand in the corresponding direction.

Of course, some people can't see the top of the chart even when they're right in front of it. These people may be able to see movement,

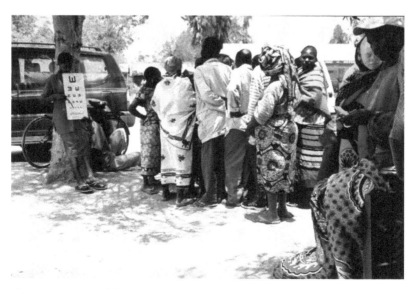

Figure 1.1 A 'tumbling-E' Snellen chart being used to test vision in Tanzania. H Kuper. Attribution-NonCommercial 4.0 International (CC BY-NC 4.0). Image from: https://wellcomecollection.org/works/hzyjwfpq.

colours or lights and this vision can still be useful. The difference between being able to see daylight through a window and not seeing anything at all can have a huge impact on quality of life. Only a small proportion of people described as blind have no light perception at all, and even these people may sense light in different ways.

In the low vision clinic, we don't use Snellen charts, as they are not the most accurate way to measure visual acuity in people with vision impairment. There are very few letters towards the top of the chart with big gaps between the letter sizes, so quite large changes in vision cannot always be detected. The larger letters are shown on their own rather than as a row of characters, which makes them easier to identify, and it's quite easy to accidentally memorise the first few letters on the chart. Instead we tend to use logarithmic letter charts, which can be shown at any distance and easily moved to an appropriate place for the person to read them.

Sam read the top line of the chart when I wheeled it to half of its normal distance, meaning she had a visual acuity of 3/60, about 20 times poorer than mine. Would this mean she should be called 'blind'? The World Health Organization curates the International Classification of Diseases system, now in its eleventh iteration (the ICD-11).[3] This classification usually makes the news when new diseases are added to it, such as when hoarding disorder was added to the database, under the disease code 6B24. The ICD-11 classifies vision impairment in terms of visual acuity, ranging from 'no visual impairment' for people who see better than 6/12 (that is, anyone whose vision is good enough to allow them to drive, in most countries) through to 'blindness'. Sam's level of vision does – just – put her into the 'blind' category, so strictly speaking she would meet this definition. Table 1.1 shows the ICD-11 classification for different levels of visual acuity along with the threshold to receive a certificate of vision impairment in the UK, as sight impaired (which used to be called 'partially sighted') and severely sight impaired (formerly 'blind').[4]

As the table shows, there are people who have mild or moderate vision impairment but do not meet the threshold for registration as sight impaired. This is not unique to the UK, as the threshold for 'legal blindness' does not vary considerably around the world, with most countries using the same criterion as 'sight impairment' in the UK (although in India the level is equivalent to the British 'severely sight impaired' level).[5] Someone with moderate vision impairment normally would not be allowed to drive, may well use magnifiers to read and may need mobility training to navigate safely, but would not receive

Table 1.1 Levels of vision impairment defined by the ICD-11[1] and corresponding levels of UK certification of vision impairment.[2]

Level of vision	ICD-11 definition	Certificate of visual impairment
Better than 6/12	No vision impairment	Not eligible
6/12 to 6/18 *2–3 times poorer than good vision*	Mild vision impairment	Not eligible
6/18 to 6/60 *3–10 times poorer than good vision*	Moderate vision impairment	Not eligible
6/60 to 3/60 *10–20 times poorer than good vision*	Severe vision impairment	Sight impairment
Worse than 3/60, including light perception and no light perception; OR visual field of <10° radius	Blindness	Severe sight impairment

[1] World Health Organization. ICD-11: International Classification of Diseases (11th Revision). 2019. http://who.int.

[2] Department of Health. Certificate of Vision Impairment: Explanatory Notes for Consultant Ophthalmologists and Hospital Eye Clinic Staff in England, 2017. https://assets.publishing. service.gov.uk/government/uploads/system/uploads/attachment_data/file/637590/CVI_ guidance.pdf.

the help and protection associated with legal registration. This group of people is sometimes said to have 'low vision' and they may struggle to communicate their vision loss to their teachers, employers and friends, partly as they don't have the shorthand of being able to say 'I'm registered as sight impaired' or 'I'm legally blind'.

Like many people with vision impairment who don't wear spectacles, Sam sometimes gets asked: 'Can't you get glasses to help you see better?' Leaving aside the ignorance of this question (do people really think that she wouldn't have thought of that?), it's important to note that for these purposes vision is measured with glasses on and with both eyes open. For the same reason, the people who try and empathise with Sam by saying 'I'm blind without my glasses' miss the point, as if they can see well with their glasses on and they have access to the correct spectacles (sadly not the case in much of the world, as we shall see later), they are not vision impaired.

Visual field

The other measurement I consider when I'm assessing how well someone sees is their visual field, which is how much of the world they can see at once, without moving their eyes. You can check this yourself at home by staring at something straight ahead (something small, like a light switch, is ideal), holding your left arm out as if you're signalling to turn left on a bicycle, pushing your arm back as far as it will go, wiggling your fingers, then moving your arm forward slowly. You should first see your fingers moving when your arm is about level with your shoulder.

To quantify this measurement, you can think about the angle between the direction you are looking and the angle of your arm (Figure 1.2). This angle is about 90 degrees, so your visual field extends around 90 degrees to that side of your eye. If you do something similar with your arm in front of you, you can measure the vertical extent of your visual field. Someone with a full visual field can probably see about 80 degrees down without moving their eyes, which is useful for detecting obstacles and steps. The visual field does not extend quite so far upwards, usually reaching only about 70 degrees, a fact lamented by anyone who has banged their head on a low doorframe or cycled into an overhanging branch.

Measuring visual fields precisely is more difficult than asking someone to hold their arms out and wave them around as if they are directing traffic. You may have noticed it was difficult to keep your eyes still when you were doing this test, as it is natural to try and peek towards where your hand is. Modern visual field tests monitor the position of the eyes. These machines look like large bowls which the patient puts their head into, like a miniature planetarium. A spot of light will flash at various places around the bowl and the patient presses a button when the light is seen. It can be a tedious test for patient and practitioner alike. Kurt Vonnegut's *Slaughterhouse Five*[6] includes a scene where an

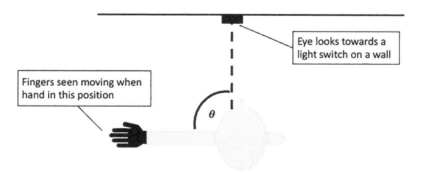

Eye looks towards a
light switch on a wall

Fingers seen moving when
hand in this position

θ

Figure 1.2   A top-down view of a way to approximately measure the visual field. Angle θ shows the extent of the visual field to the left. Image drawn by the author.

optometrist falls asleep in the middle of an eye examination (the only example of an optometrist hero in literature that I am aware of). I would be willing to bet this scenario happened when the lights were dimmed for a visual field test.

Visual field loss results from many eye diseases and can happen independently of visual acuity loss. It's not uncommon for me to meet people in the clinic who can read letters on the bottom line of the chart but who have a visual field of only a couple of degrees, as if they are looking at the world through a drinking straw. It may take them several seconds to find where the vision chart is, even in an uncluttered room, and they may need to be guided to the chair. If I ask them to look at my nose, they can't see my eyes or mouth without moving their eyes around and they tell me they are frequently surprised by someone suddenly appearing in front of them. They are likely to struggle with mobility and may well use a white cane or have a guide dog. People with severe visual field loss meet the image that most people have of 'a blind person' and the ICD-11 recognises this by classifying anyone with a visual field of less than 10 degrees as 'blind'.

The most common cause of visual field loss is glaucoma, a group of diseases where the eye's nerve fibres stop functioning, often because the pressure in the eye is too high. In glaucoma people tend to lose their peripheral vision over a period of years. This gradually increasing tunnel vision is very difficult for the person to notice, but once visual field is lost in glaucoma it normally cannot be recovered. This is one of the main reasons why it's important for people to have their eyes examined regularly, so the visual field can be checked to screen for glaucoma, the so-called 'thief of sight'. Glaucoma is more common in older people and in some populations, such as Black African people. Once diagnosed, the progression of visual field loss can usually be slowed or stopped with an operation or by using eye drops.

Tunnel vision is not the only type of field loss. Sam's eye condition affected her central retina so, although she could see well to the sides, she had a blind spot right in the middle of her vision, blocking her view of anything she looked at directly. Age-related macular disease causes a similar central field loss, whereas stroke and brain injury can cause hemianopia, which is an absence of exactly half of the visual field.

Although visual acuity and visual field are the most significant measures of vision, there are other factors that are relevant when thinking about how well someone sees. The ability to recognise colours and to see well under different light levels is also important. Contrast sensitivity is another key part of how well someone sees. People with reduced contrast

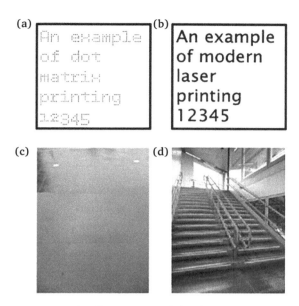

(a) An example of dot matrix printing 12345

(b) An example of modern laser printing 12345

(c)

(d)

Figure 1.3 An example of low-contrast (left column) and high-contrast (right column) tasks. Images drawn/photographed by the author.

sensitivity can see black on white objects quite well but struggle with grey print on a grey background. These people often tell me that many websites are designed with 'young eyes' in mind, with thin grey writing against an off-white background. When I teach trainees about contrast sensitivity, I have stopped talking about dot matrix printers (they smile and nod at me like I did as a child when an older neighbour talked to me about the Second World War), but these printouts were particularly troublesome for people with poor contrast (Figure 1.3a and 1.3b).

Not being able to see subtle changes in contrast is also important for mobility. Identifying the edge of a concrete step in the rain on a grey day can be difficult even for people with perfect sight, but can be impossible for people with reduced contrast sensitivity (Figure 1.3c). This is why steps should have high-contrast markers at their edges, as found on the London Underground (Figure 1.3d).

There are other functional ways to describe vision loss. In 1920, the UK's Blind Persons Act used an employment-based definition, stating that people were blind if they were 'so blind as to be unable to perform any work for which eyesight is essential'.[7] A functional definition of low vision is to be 'unable to read a newspaper with conventional glasses'.[8] Almost every organisation seems to have its own preferred definition, each of which includes a different proportion of the world's population.

What causes blindness?

Only a small proportion of people are born with no sight at all, usually because the visual parts of the brain are severely damaged, or because they are born without fully developed eyes. Others are born with inherited conditions such as albinism, where vision is reduced but stable throughout life. Some, like Sam, start noticing poor vision in their teens, but the overwhelming majority of people with vision impairment lose their sight later in life.

More than half of the people with significant vision impairment in most high-income countries have age-related macular degeneration (AMD). The macula is the central part of the retina, which is the most sensitive to detail and which is used to look straight at something. In the most common 'dry' form of AMD, cells in the macula gradually die, reducing central vision over many years. In contrast, in the neovascular or 'wet' type of age-related macular degeneration, new blood vessels quickly grow into the macula and leak, leading to a sudden drop in vision. For about 10 years, wet AMD has been treatable with drugs injected into the eye, stopping the growth of these blood vessels and causing them to regress. Dry macular degeneration remains untreatable, although it may be slowed by lifestyle changes such as stopping smoking and by adopting a Mediterranean diet of vegetables, fruits, legumes, cereals, fish and moderate amounts of alcohol, while also limiting meat and dairy consumption. Age-related macular disease is remarkably common in older adults. One in eight people over 80 years old in the UK have lost vision due to AMD.[9]

Glaucoma is the second most common cause of severe sight impairment in Europe and is responsible for many cases of blindness in the Global South and middle-income countries, largely because of lack of access to treatment. However, the biggest cause of severe vision loss worldwide is cataract, where the lens within the eye becomes opaque. Usually associated with age (a former colleague used to tell his patients that everyone with grey hair has a bit of cataract), in high-income countries cataracts are treated with a routine 20-minute operation. Despite the relative simplicity of this procedure, it still requires a clean operating theatre, implantable lenses and a skilled surgeon. There are about 3,000 ophthalmologists in the UK for a population of 65 million, but in Somalia there is only one ophthalmologist for every 2.5 million people.[10] This inequality of access to surgery is a major reason why more than 10 million people around the world are blind from cataracts.[11]

Even more shocking is the number of people who simply don't have spectacles. More than 100 million people are visually impaired because they do not have access to the correct glasses.[12] My smartphone tells me that I can get spectacles made in more than 20 different opticians' practices within a mile of my office in central London. I can be confident that they will be prescribed correctly and, if I had low income, the NHS would pay for the eye examination and glasses. In much of the Global South, it is impossible to access any eye care at all, and even the US$3 cost of a cheap pair of glasses is prohibitive to many.[13]

Optometrists, ophthalmologists and others

I have already mentioned optometrists and ophthalmologists so it might be useful here to define the many different people who work in the eye clinic, nearly all of whom have a job title which starts with the letter O.

I am an optometrist, which literally means an 'eye-measurer'. The bulk of my optometry degree was spent studying the physics and biology of vision, alongside some clinical skills teaching. Most of my peers from university went on to work in high-street optometry practices, measuring vision, prescribing glasses and contact lenses, detecting serious eye disease and treating minor eye conditions. I didn't follow them into primary care, instead finishing my training in an eye hospital as part of a team working with people with severe eye disease. My PhD investigated changes in eye movements made by people with macular disease, then I specialised in working in the low vision clinic, where I see people like Sam and assess their vision using all the tests described above. Like my optometrist colleagues in the community, I prescribe spectacles, but also dispense low vision aids like high-power glasses, telescopes, magnifying glasses and specialist tinted lenses. I demonstrate high-tech electronic devices and give advice on techniques to use the eyes more effectively, such as how to make eye movements to overcome visual field loss. Perhaps most importantly, I make sure that people with vision impairment are supported by all the other services they need. I can refer them to a huge range of other professionals, from counsellors to specialist teachers, all within the same hospital. On my clinic days, I spend the morning in a children's low vision clinic and the afternoon working with adults, which means I might assess a four-year-old and someone who is 104 on the same day.

All the patients I see will also visit the clinic of an ophthalmologist, a medical doctor specialising in eye disease. Ophthalmology training is tough – it takes at least six years of specialist training after medical school – and very competitive, perhaps as it is a nice specialism to work in, with few night shifts, generally healthy patients and the ability to have a big impact on people's quality of life.

I also work with orthoptists (specialists in eye movements and children's vision), ophthalmic nurses, dispensing opticians (who fit and make spectacles), ocularists (who make false eyes) and ophthalmic technicians. Beyond the jobs starting with the letter 'O', I work with specialist teachers of vision impairment, eye clinic liaison officers, counsellors, play specialists, paediatricians, medical photographers and clinic clerks. A colleague at Royal Dutch Visio (a specialist charity for people with sight loss) once told me that they employed people from 18 different professions to support their clients.

Sam didn't call her band 'Legally Blind' in the end. She is proud to define herself as a Londoner, a student, a vegan, a punk singer and a central midfielder, and she considers vision loss to be the least interesting thing about her.

Notes

1   Kuusisto, 1998.
2   Kleege, 1999.
3   World Health Organization, 2019.
4   Department of Health, 2017.
5   KV and Vijayalakshmi, 2020.
6   Vonnegut, 1970.
7   Dickinson, 1998.
8   Leat, 2011.
9   Owen et al., 2012.
10   Resnikoff et al., 2020.
11   Khairallah et al., 2015.
12   Adelson et al., 2021.
13   Durr et al., 2014.

2
Swallowed by darkness: art and vision impairment

Artist Luka Kille shudders when she tells me about being forced as a teenager to explain her visual impairment to her classmates. A well-meaning teacher had brought a big box of simulation spectacles to her school, so that her school friends could experience what her vision was like:

> They were all like, 'Oh my God, this is so horrible, I feel so sorry for Luka.' It was terrible for me, it was so awful, I felt pity and it was really bad … then I tried some on myself and I was like, 'This is not even what I see, this is nothing like what my experience is like'… it's boiling my entire experience down to only the things that don't work.

Luka emphasises what she *can* see, rather than what she can't, throughout our conversation. She describes her vision loss in artistic terms, saying that her view of the world is like a photorealistic painting, rather than the high-definition photographic image of someone with perfect vision:

> I see everything. I see things that are beautiful, I see landscapes. If you look at a painting you can see everything, but you might not be able to see the detail, and that's how I like to put it. It's not disrupted in a way that is necessarily bad or really scary – it's different. There's less visual information but it's smooth; things are quite tolerable in general. It's like an Instagram filter.

With both eyes open Luka's vision is 6/60, which means she can only read the top letter of a sight chart from the usual distance. You might not appreciate that she is severely visually impaired from listening to her description, but if you were a 14-year-old girl losing your vision, wouldn't you rather your friends thought that you saw the world through a soft-focus filter, rather than only being able to see one-tenth as well as everyone else in the class?

Luka has been visually impaired since her teens, but is conscious that her experience as a young adult with retinal disease is not representative of everyone with visual impairment.

To broaden her knowledge of sight loss, Luka blindfolded herself completely for eight full days. The art she created based on this experience is striking, showing stark monochrome images of clouds, ladders and dark skies. The names of the pictures tell their own story. Looking at an image is almost redundant when you learn it is called 'Head in the cloud. Connected yet distant. Out of touch.'

My favourite picture in the series is the title piece of the collection, 'Daring into darkness' (Figure 2.1). A ladder breaks through a starry sky, extending off the top of the image. Luka told me this drawing reflects the absence of walls when she was blindfolded:

> I didn't really perceive walls or spaces the same way. I felt like it was opening up my sense of internal and external, because all of a sudden I could hear birds outside ... usually we are visually focused on our surroundings and limited by the walls we are within, within one floor, within one room. When you don't have that visual wall, you just perceive the room and the dimensions very differently.

Another piece, titled 'Time loses meaning. My body beats at a new rhythm now, out of time with the world. Calm' (Figure 2.2), shows clocks spiralling into the distance. Luka missed being able to judge time by looking at the sky, that 'shortcut orientation of where you're at in the cycle of your day', as she puts it. Some blind people feel that they are so out of rhythm with the passing of time that they take the sleep hormone melatonin every evening, to help their body differentiate night from day.

Luka didn't rely on technology when she was blindfolded, despite being familiar with accessibility features on computers and smartphones. In particular, the VoiceOver feature on her phone, which reads messages and emails aloud, didn't suit her as she found the voice startling and the overall effect disruptive. After three days she abandoned her devices, focusing instead on the world around her.

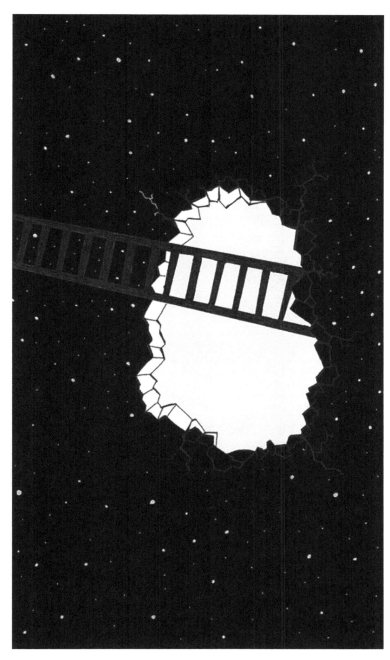

Figure 2.1 'Daring into darkness' by Luka Kille, 2017. Reproduced with kind permission of the artist.

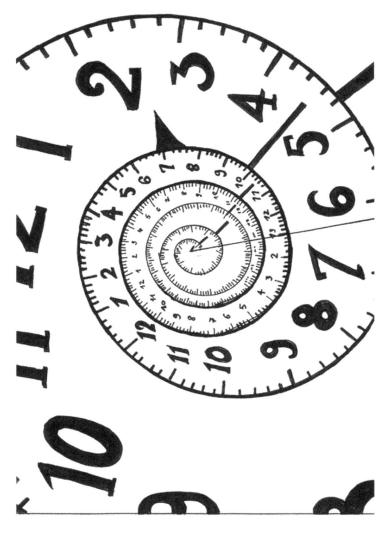

Figure 2.2 'Time loses meaning. My body beats at a new rhythm now, out of time with the world. Calm' by Luka Kille, 2017. Reproduced with kind permission of the artist.

Luka is a successful artist, having studied at the Royal College of Art and exhibited her work around Europe. This might surprise the careers teacher she met at school, who told her that art would not be in her future. After initially being upset by this conversation, Luka took inspiration from another artist with visual impairment: 'Somehow Monet's paintings helped me accept my fate and my vision … I said (to myself): "No, you're not right, in fact it might make your art more interesting, like in Monet's case."'

Claude Monet's sequential paintings of the Japanese bridge at Giverny, in France, show the effects of cataracts growing in his eyes, with the colours and definition becoming less clear over time. A cataract is an opacification of the lens inside the eye. In its early stages, it reduces the amount of light that gets to the retina, making the world dimmer and less vivid. At the same time, a cataract causes light to scatter around the eye, making it difficult to see in bright light. Today, the commonest early sign of a cataract developing is difficulty with driving at night, when light from oncoming headlights hits the opacities in the lens, dazzling the driver's view of the road.

In Monet's time, cataract surgery was a far more dangerous endeavour than it is today, and operations were deferred until the cataracts were 'ripe', by which time the lens would be yellow or brown, so the entire world would appear dark and nicotine-stained. This colour shift makes blue difficult to see, and makes white objects look red or yellow.

Monet's cataracts are perhaps the most famous in the art world, but it is even easier to see the colour shift associated with cataract in the work of Edgar Degas. Compare Degas' 1883 painting 'Woman in a Tub' to his 'Woman at her Toilet' 11 years later (Figures 2.3 and 2.4). The later work is redder, less detailed and darker, which is exactly the shift that would be expected from seeing the world through a cataract.

Retrospectively diagnosing artists' eye disease is a passion for some ophthalmologists. In his 1970 book *The World through Blunted Sight*, ophthalmologist Patrick Trevor-Roper described the impact of vision loss on dozens of artists.[1] Trevor-Roper sounds like a fascinating man. As well as being an ophthalmologist and author, he was an early advocate for gay rights, was involved in the founding of the HIV charity, the Terrence Higgins Trust, and campaigned against drug companies sponsoring medical conferences. I am sad not to have met him, as he retired before I qualified, but his achievements are commemorated in a portrait on the ground floor of Moorfields Eye Hospital in London.

As well as looking for evidence of severe visual impairment in the work of famous artists, Trevor-Roper explored which artists might have

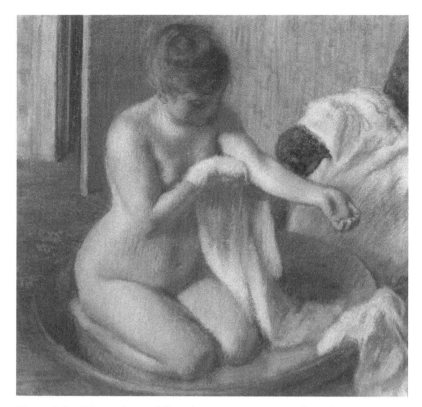

Figure 2.3 'Woman in a Tub' by Edgar Degas, c. 1883. Wikimedia Commons. Public domain.

needed glasses but didn't wear them. He spent time photographing famous paintings through various spectacle lenses, investigating whether an uncorrected need for glasses could explain the appearance of some major works. This phenomenon seems to have been particularly widespread amongst the Impressionists. Paul Cézanne refused to wear glasses (apparently saying 'take those vulgar things away' when offered some), as did Pierre-Auguste Renoir, who reportedly said 'Good God, I see like Bouguereau' when he tried glasses. William-Adolphe Bouguereau was a conventional naturalistic painter of the period, clearly not appreciated by Renoir.

Why did so many of the French Impressionists have difficulty with their eyesight? It's not impossible that their blurred vision made painting in the Impressionist style easier, but it could also be that their vision made them unfit for military service, freeing them from the Franco-Prussian War of 1870 for the more peaceful activity of painting.

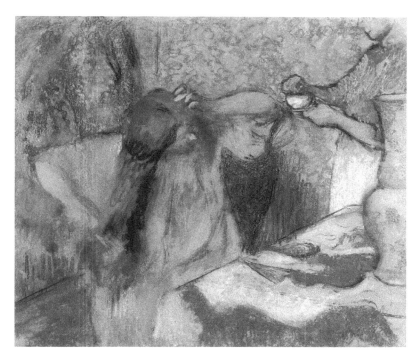

Figure 2.4   'Woman at her Toilet' by Edgar Degas, c. 1894. Public domain, via wikiart.org.

Luka had a bad experience with simulation glasses, but finding a better way of describing the world as seen by someone with vision impairment is challenging. This is a particular interest of David Crabb, Professor of Statistics and Vision Research at City, University of London. One problem with using pictures or simulation glasses is that a person with good sight can move their eyes around, to look around the simulated blind region. Professor Crabb and his group are using a virtual reality environment, complete with eye tracking, to overcome this problem and create a more accurate simulation of sight loss. In their study 'Seeing the world through someone else's eyes', they are demonstrating the impact of vision impairment on everyday visual tasks, such as finding a mobile phone.

Pictures in books that are supposed to represent different eye conditions often show the world as surrounded by black regions, or with black spots in front of the image. This is very rarely the experience of people with vision impairment. In one study of 153 people with significant loss of their central vision, only two saw a dark patch overlaying the world. For both of these people, the black area was only seen for a short time on waking, and faded after they got out of bed.[2]

One reason for this is the phenomenon of filling in, where the brain uses colours and textures from the rest of the visual field to 'paint over' any gaps in the visual field. This is the same reason why people are not aware of the blind spot that naturally occurs in every human eye, corresponding to the head of the optic nerve. Filling in means that people with sight loss tend to describe their vision as being blurred, or incomplete, or to describe the functional effects of not seeing something, rather like Sam not seeing the ketchup bottle described in the previous chapter. In Crabb's paper 'How Does Glaucoma Look?', he found that people with glaucoma tended to choose an image with blurred patches as the best simulation of what their sight was like, with none selecting a picture with a black surround or black patches on it.[3]

Sculpture

Fans of 1980s pop music may know the rather uncomfortable video for Lionel Richie's 1984 hit 'Hello', featuring Richie as an art teacher with a crush on a young blind student. His love appears to be unrequited, until in the final sequence it is revealed that the student has made a perfect sculpture of Lionel Richie's head. The video is, rightly, derided. *Mic* magazine put it on their list of '5 music videos from the '80s that prove it was the era of uncomfortable feels', pointing out that Richie and the student 'don't talk much; he just creeps up behind her in different settings'.[4] The video ends with Lionel Richie allowing the student to touch his face, an experience that is all too common for people who are blind. M. Leona Godin describes this in her book *There Plant Eyes*:

> I would have never asked to feel anyone's face, although I have had many sighted people ask if I *want* to feel their face. It always makes me laugh. I would prefer not to feel any faces out of the contexts in which most sighted people feel faces: intimate moments with loved ones such as spouses or children.[5]

Although the video for *Hello* is problematic on many levels (I've not even mentioned the teacher/student dynamic), sculpture is a form of the visual arts accessible to people with vision impairment.

Artist Lenka Clayton noticed that a sculpture by Constantin Brancusi titled 'Sculpture for the Blind' was, ironically, displayed behind glass at the Philadelphia Museum of Art. She took detailed notes about the sculpture and wrote a 240-word description of it. The description contains factual details, such as its size, the fact that 'the top of the object is a flatter, gently rounded plane' and 'except for a thin fold line on the front, shorter than a finger length, the surface is smooth and unbroken'. It also includes some poetic, emotive details: 'Like a cat, it would fit easily on your lap and would take two hands to hold comfortably,' and 'The right end is larger and appears to swell, resembling the back of a baby's head.'[6]

I wish I'd heard Clayton's description before seeing a picture of the sculpture, as it would be fascinating to compare my mental image of the sculpture with its real appearance. As part of her own artwork, Lenka read her description to a group of 17 people with vision impairment from Philadelphia and invited them to try and duplicate the sculpture by creating it themselves. The resulting set of sculptures, titled 'Sculpture for the Blind, by the Blind' shows the diversity of impressions based on the same description. In the spirit of Lenka Clayton's work, I should attempt to describe the resulting artwork in words, but I lack the artistic vocabulary to say much beyond the fact that there are 17 black tables, each with a white rock-shaped sculpture on, of varying sizes and bulginess (Figure 2.5).

The experience of not being able to touch a sculpture also frustrated Felice Tagliaferri, a visually impaired sculptor from Italy. In response to not being allowed to touch 'Cristo Velato (Veiled Christ)' by Giuseppe

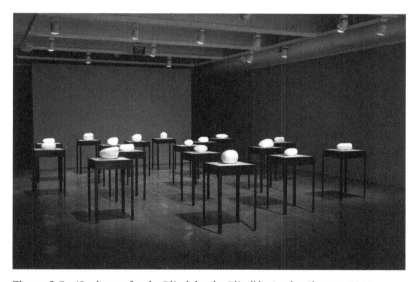

Figure 2.5 'Sculpture for the Blind, by the Blind' by Lenka Clayton, 2017. Reproduced with kind permission of the artist.

Sanmartino on a visit to Naples, Tagliaferri made an accessible version of the statue called 'Cristo Rivelato (Revealed Christ)'. He cheekily inverts the instructions found in many galleries, saying 'You are forbidden not to touch.'[7]

Luka is still able to go to galleries and see the art with the help of a low vision aid, but how is art communicated to people who have no sight? Audio description and braille notes can help, but perhaps the most intuitive way to interact with art is indeed to touch it. The charity Living Paintings provides tactile versions of images for people of all ages who have sight loss, from 'Touch to See' children's picture books on art history to tactile guides to the Royal Academy and Tate Britain.[8] One of their adult users, who has been visually impaired since birth, says that he was initially apprehensive – 'I thought art was very posh and only for the upper classes and very visual. Why on earth would you show paintings to a blind guy?' – but now says he has learnt a huge amount about art, 'as well as discovering beautiful works of art through touch'.[9]

In the same report, a teacher of visual impairment explains how accessing art can help a child with low vision understand the world: 'When my student read [the popular children's book] *Handa's Surprise* and looked very closely at the illustration of the elephant, she said "Oh, is that what an elephant looks like, I didn't know."' These books are also helpful for blind parents of children with good sight, who can use embossed pictures to talk about the books with their children. Alba, a parent with no sight, explains what this involves: 'I now read to Eliot every evening, he sits on my lap and listens, and then he takes my hand and shows me the pictures and we talk about them together.'[9]

Touch tours exist in several galleries, although it is rare for museums to allow anyone to touch their most priceless works. Georgina Kleege is an American writer who lost her sight at the age of 11 and whose parents were both (sighted) artists. In her book *More than Meets the Eye: What blindness brings to art*, she writes:

> Incidentally, it has been my experience that artists are a lot less squeamish about letting people touch their work than are art conservators. Without name-dropping, I admit here that my finger-prints are all over any number of mid-twentieth-century art on display in museums and private collections around the world.[10]

Other galleries have experimented with incorporating music, smell and even taste to help visitors with reduced vision interact with their art works.[11]

Art doesn't only exist in formal galleries, as most towns and cities are full of murals, graffiti walls and statues. In India, the right to access art is enshrined in law, with the Rights of Persons with Disabilities Act 2016 ensuring that art and culture is accessible for recreational as well as educational and professional purposes. Ishan Chakraborty, a Professor of English at Jadavpur University in Kolkata who has vision impairment, has ensured that this right extends to street art. With his students, he has used bisected table tennis balls to create 'braille graffiti'. He writes that the aim of the project was to promote communication between people with good vision and those with vision impairment, as well as raising understanding that 'access to art is not a luxury and should not be treated as such'.[12]

Architecture

In the low vision clinic, we use the mantra of 'big, bright and bold' to help amateur artists paint. The view of their canvas can be enlarged with telescopic magnifiers; optimal lighting makes the painting brighter and more visible; and appropriate colour contrast makes art materials easier to see (red paint stands out best on a white palette, but light colours are more visible against a black mixing tray). It is common for people to continue with their hobby using these adaptations. In fact, I have seen many people who start painting after being diagnosed with a sight-threatening condition, perhaps due to a newfound appreciation of the visual world, or as a way to capture what can still be seen. But what happens if someone who works in the visual arts abruptly loses all of their sight?

At the age of 45, having been an architect for nearly 20 years, Chris Downey had emergency surgery to remove a brain tumour. The operation saved his life but left him completely blind, with no perception of light in either eye. Amazingly, Downey was back at work within a month of losing his sight. He has since worked on several flagship public buildings around the world, including the sustainability pavilion at Expo 2020 Dubai, a charity headquarters in San Francisco and the University of Pittsburgh Medical Center. In an interview with *Interior Design* magazine, Chris says that losing his vision has made him a better architect:

> I tend to think of my sight loss as completing my architectural training. I used to obsess on the visual aspects of architecture.

Losing my sight taught me to think about architecture in more multisensory ways and to think about how a broad range of people experience design – whether it's visually, through sound, or by walking through a space.[13]

Chris talks about using non-visual cues to mark transitions between different areas of a building, so embossed floor markings indicate the start of a staircase, or carpets surround reception desks so that the start of the reception area can be felt and heard as well as seen. He rejects the idea of being a blind architect as unusual – after all, no architect can physically see their buildings before they are complete. Speaking on the fascinating podcast *99% Invisible*, Downey says:

> Beethoven continued to write music and wrote some of his best music after he lost his hearing, so he couldn't hear his music at all; he could only hear the construction in his mind. And as architects we have all sorts of different ways of experiencing architecture both in its built form and its creation through tactile drawings and models besides our own mental constructions.[14]

I discussed tactile drawings and some other adaptations with Shital, a second-year architecture student who was starting to lose his sight due to an optic nerve disease:

'That's fine if you're Chris Downey, who was already a partner with a massive team,' Shital said. 'But it's so tough applying for jobs anyway … if I go in and say "I need you to use tactile drawings and you need to make models at an earlier stage" they'll say "Sorry, but we've already got our intern for this year."'

Instead, Shital relies on another mainstay of the architect's office – the huge Mac monitor – which he can just about see from a few centimetres away using strong glasses.

'I don't know, I guess I'd rather start off doing it the same as everyone else,' he told me. 'If things get worse, I'll think again, but I can manage for now. It takes me longer, but I still love it.'

For school students, vision impairment doesn't seem to be a major barrier to enjoying art lessons. I always ask children in the low vision clinic what their favourite lesson is. Art is high up the list, although 'lunchtime' is still the most common answer to 'What's your favourite thing at school?' Depending on the type of vision loss they have, I might ask whether they have difficulty recognising colours, seeing fine details or reproducing things they see. It is rare for me to hear any concerns about this, perhaps as art is so adaptable – there is always a thicker brush, a darker pen or a more Impressionist style to adopt. It appears that art teachers are some of the most understanding school staff at accepting different methods of expressing yourself. Art is, after all, about your personal interpretation of the world.

Film

If I ask someone to picture a blind person, they often imagine a character they have seen on film, usually being played by an actor with good sight who uses cultural tropes to determine how a person with vision impairment should behave. In her excellent 1999 book *Sight Unseen*, Georgina Kleege divides blind film characters into those who are 'morose, cranky, resentful, socially awkward and prone to despair', and those who are 'blind seers'.[15] This second trope is typified by the character Zatōichi, an itinerant blind swordsman who is the hero of one of Japan's longest-running film franchises, appearing in 26 films and a 100-episode TV series. The standard Zatōichi story is that he arrives in a small village, meets the locals when drinking or gambling, discovers an injustice, then rights the wrongs by his expert use of a samurai sword (which, symbolically, he hides inside his mobility cane). This knight errant story isn't new or unusual – it's been exploited by Lee Child to sell millions of Jack Reacher novels – but I do wonder whether the popularity of Zatōichi in Japan means that blind people there are perceived slightly differently.

Kleege highlights that actors are generally very poor at portraying vision-impaired characters, writing that 'most blind people are better at appearing sighted than the sighted are at appearing blind'. I haven't seen all the films which she discusses and recommend her book for a detailed description of 'blind cinema', but I would like to present two examples of film characters with vision impairment as I think these represent the two extremes of how blind people are shown on screen.

The blind character I find least realistic is one which seems to have been most widely seen: Al Pacino's performance in the 1992 film *Scent of a Woman*. Pacino plays Frank Slade, a misogynistic, alcoholic, retired army Lieutenant Colonel, blinded in the Vietnam War. When his family are travelling, they employ a naïve student (Charlie, played by Chris O'Donnell) to look after Slade, little knowing that the retired soldier will bully Charlie into taking a trip to New York, where they stay in a luxury hotel and attempt to pick up women. Pacino's character perpetuates multiple stereotypes of blindness, including a superpower (the frankly creepy ability to recognise a woman's perfume and soap brands alluded to in the film's title) and inappropriate behaviour (grabby hands, moral laxity, behaviour which endangers others) which is broadly tolerated 'because he's blind'. Most disturbingly, the film centres on an unquestioned assumption that taking your own life is a reasonable response to losing your sight.

Far fewer films show blind people as normal, flawed, angry, happy people. My favourite portrayal of a vision-impaired character by a sighted actor is in Lars von Trier's 2000 film *Dancer in the Dark*. The Icelandic singer and artist Björk plays Selma Ježková, an Eastern European migrant working in a factory in Washington state in the 1960s. Selma has a progressive, inherited eye disease which causes severe vision impairment. Selma knows, but her son doesn't, that he has inherited the same gene, so Selma saves all the money she can to pay for a potential future treatment for her son. She disguises her vision loss at work, risking serious injury, and lies to her ophthalmologist about how well she sees by memorising the sight charts shown to her. I found Selma very believable and liked the fact that her blindness was a plot device rather than being the whole centrepiece of the film – it's more about crime, family, truth and the death penalty than vision impairment. When I asked Georgina Kleege what she thought of this portrayal, she admitted that since researching her book she has avoided watching any movies with a blind character. As she writes in *Sight Unseen*: 'If I want to have nightmares I go to movies about the blind.'[15]

As far as I know, Björk has good vision. Should her role have been played by a blind actor? The National Federation of the Blind in the USA recently protested outside the CBS office in Manhattan over their TV production *In the Dark* which used sighted actors to play blind characters. One of the placards read 'Let us play us,' echoing earlier protests around 'blacking up' and current debates over whether heterosexual actors should play gay characters.[16]

I am not aware of any protests around *Dancer in the Dark*, but it divided reviewers for other reasons. The film has an unusual structure. It is bleak and brutal, but interspersed with imaginary upbeat musical interludes. One of these musical numbers is 'I've Seen it All', written by Björk and Thom Yorke. In this song, Selma's friend Jeff laments the things that she will never see. In a display of (mock?) acceptance, Selma underplays not having experienced these things visually:

Jeff: What about China? Have you seen the Great Wall?
Selma: All walls are great if the roof doesn't fall.

Jeff: And the man you will marry?
The home you will share?
Selma: To be honest, I really don't care …

Jeff: You've never been to Niagara Falls?
Selma: I have seen water, it's water, that's all …
Björk. *I've Seen It All*; One Little Independent Records: London, 2000.[17]

Audio description is available for most films, many plays and some TV productions. By wearing headphones, the person with vision impairment hears a description of the visual action on the screen ('the woman with grey hair looks angrily at the child playing with the toys'). It doesn't always work well, particularly for subtitled films, although I recently heard a very favourable review of the audio description offered at London's National Theatre. Not everyone with mild or moderate vision impairment needs this level of description, particularly at the cinema, where the large and colourful screen exemplifies 'big, bright and bold'.

Music

It would be difficult to write about music and visual impairment without mentioning Stevie Wonder, perhaps the most famous blind person of the twentieth century. Stevie Wonder was born, two months prematurely, in May 1950. Doctors kept him alive by placing him in an incubator with a high concentration of oxygen. At that time, the effect of high doses of oxygen on tiny babies wasn't fully understood. In Wonder's case, it led to a rapid and uncontrolled growth of blood vessels in his still developing eyes, causing retinal detachment and lifelong vision impairment. This condition, initially given the tongue-twisting name retrolental fibroplasia, but now more commonly called retinopathy of prematurity, or ROP, became widespread in high-income countries in the 1950s as doctors got better at helping preterm babies survive. As awareness of ROP became more widespread, neonatal doctors started using less oxygen in preterm babies, which led to fewer cases of blindness, but an increase in cerebral palsy and in children not surviving.[18] More recent research suggests that supplemental oxygen isn't the only cause of ROP, as some premature babies develop the condition without receiving any extra oxygen being given.[19] To reduce the amount of blindness associated with ROP, every baby at risk of developing the disease (particularly those who weigh less than 1,500 grams at birth and those who were born before 30 weeks) should be examined by an ophthalmologist. In most cases of ROP the disease regresses as the baby grows, but in some cases laser treatment, drugs to limit blood vessel growth or retinal surgery are needed. These treatments are so successful that the World Health Organization now classifies ROP as a preventable cause of blindness.[20]

It is rare for me to see children with ROP in the low vision clinic, but I still see people of Stevie Wonder's generation who have lived with this condition for their whole life. They are often very short-sighted and have retinal problems affecting their visual field. Some, like Stevie Wonder, are unable to perceive any light at all.

Much like the punk songs written by Sam in Chapter 1, Stevie Wonder's music doesn't often reference his sight loss, but he does advocate for the blind community. On his 1972 album *Talking Book* (itself a reference to a major leisure activity for people with vision impairment), he included a braille inscription, reading 'Here is my music. It is all that I have to tell you how I feel. Know that your love keeps me strong – Stevie.'[21] This action was not appreciated by his record label, as the extra thickness of the record cover meant they could put 20 per cent fewer albums into a crate, or onto a record shop's shelf.

Many years later, the US Treasury Department successfully used the same argument when opposing tactile markings on American dollar banknotes. Unlike most currencies, where larger notes correspond to higher values, all American banknotes are the same size. They also have minimal colour coding, making them almost impossible to differentiate without good sight. A raised feature would allow people to identify the value of each note by touch, but the extra thickness would have added an unacceptable extra cost to the vending industry and problems in stacking banknotes. Subsequent lawsuits have made the development of more accessible dollar notes inevitable, although perhaps not before electronic payments have replaced the use of cash.

On Stevie Wonder's next album, *Innervisions*, there is an allusion to sight loss in the song 'Living for the City'. The middle section of the full-length version of this track contains a minute-long audio picture of New York. Sounds overlap and oscillate between the left and right ear: traffic, sirens, street hustlers, racist police officers and finally a courtroom judge. The soundscape involves a naïve out-of-towner stepping off a coach in the middle of the city, being hustled, wrongly arrested, tried and imprisoned. It's stunningly evocative, recreating street life so well that I can almost imagine the smell of diesel fumes when listening to it. The authenticity is helped by the use of genuine cops who ad-libbed their lines, while the anger which you hear in Wonder's voice is real as his band re-recorded and re-recorded the vocal until Stevie was tired, hoarse and deeply annoyed.[21] At the song's launch, Stevie Wonder arranged for journalists to be driven around the city blindfolded, to experience the city as he does.[22]

The sounds of New York City also influenced the blind musician Moondog. A successful composer, writing music for Janis Joplin and others, Moondog was best known for busking on Sixth Avenue in Manhattan in the 1940s, wearing a cape and a Viking-style horned hat and selling books of poetry. His compositions are influenced by the sounds which surrounded him in New York like the rumble of trains, blasts of foghorns and intermittent episodes of birdsong. His most famous song, 'Bird's Lament', can still be heard on the radio and in TV adverts, particularly in its remixed version 'Get a Move On!' by Mr Scruff.

Stevie Wonder's father was largely absent and possibly abusive, but nurtured his son's musical talent by giving him a set of bongo drums before he could even walk. This was a great present. Child psychologists who specialise in vision impairment emphasise that it is important to 'bring the other senses alive' for children without vision as early use of touch-based and audio toys encourages development and reduces the chance of a blind child developing 'tactile avoidance' later in life.[23]

This advice was also followed by the parents of pianist Nobuyuki Tsujii, who has microphthalmia, meaning that he was born with very small, underdeveloped eyes. Some people with microphthalmia can see quite well, although their smaller eyes tend to be highly long-sighted, but others, like Nobuyuki, have no perception of light at all. Tsujii's parents noticed his musical aptitude when he was eight months old, when they noticed him kicking his feet in time to a Chopin piece playing on the radio. When he was two years old, they bought him a toy piano and 30 years later he is a professional pianist who performs and records piano concertos all over the world. When asked how he stays in time without seeing the conductor, Tsujii has said, 'By listening to the conductor's breath and also sensing what's happening around me.'[24]

Technology helps Tsujii when composing, with software that transcribes whatever he plays onto a musical score, but these options were not available to the twentieth-century composer Frederick Delius, who lost most of his vision due to syphilis, a relatively common cause of blindness before the widespread use of antibiotics. On hearing about Delius' vision loss, the young composer Eric Fenby volunteered to work as his amanuensis, someone who transcribes spoken compositions into musical notation. In his book *Delius as I Knew Him*, Fenby highlights how technically demanding this would have been:

> I want you to imagine that we are sitting on the cliffs in the heather looking out over the sea. The sustained chords in the high strings suggest the clear sky … Bring the bassoons down a semitone in thirds on the last beat, and give the cellos and basses the same rhythm as the bar before the strong chord – sings it – 'ter-ter, ter-ter'.[25]

Literature

Eric Fenby was clearly highly skilled at taking musical dictation, but an amanuensis usually works with writers, transcribing poetry or prose. The history of blind writers and their amanuenses, from Homer to Milton to James Joyce, would fill several books and I will leave it to experts in literary criticism to describe the effect of dictation on writing style. However, I will write about one of my favourite late twentieth-century writers, who became blind towards the end of her career: Sue Townsend, best known for writing a series of books about the hapless but well-intentioned Adrian Mole.

The Secret Diary of Adrian Mole (aged 13¾) was the UK's best-selling fiction book of the 1980s and continued with seven sequels, charting Adrian's life until his mid-forties. As she wrote these books, diabetes caused Townsend to go from having perfect sight to being, as she put it, 'three-quarters blind'. Initially her vision loss was subtle: 'Colours faded and my chair crept closer to the telly. My husband began to read aloud the subtitles of foreign films.'[26]

She later experienced a sudden drop in her vision, due to a retinal haemorrhage. This was at about the same time as she was organising the television adaptation of one of her books, starring Stephen Mangan. As part of the audition process, Sue Townsend peered at Mangan's face through a large magnifying glass designed for reading. In a TV documentary, Mangan recalls that 'she came right up to my face. She said "Adrian can't be too good looking." She scanned me all over … obviously I was ugly enough to play him.'[27]

Adrian Mole didn't go blind in parallel with Sue Townsend, but his best friend Nigel did. Always self-absorbed, Adrian laments the impact of Nigel's sight loss on his own life: 'I was very shocked. I had been hoping that Nigel would help me decorate my loft apartment. He used to be good with colours.'

It is tempting to think that Townsend used Nigel's character to express some of her own frustrations about living with vision impairment. Here is Adrian speaking on Nigel's behalf:

> I helped him into the cab and told the driver to take him to 5 Bill Gates Close, The Homestead Estate, near Glenfield. Nigel said in a bad-tempered way, 'I can still speak, Moley!' I hope he is not going to become one of those bitter blind people, like Mr Rochester in *Jane Eyre*.

Towards the end of her life, Townsend used a white cane, dictated her writing onto audio cassette and used an electronic magnifier to slowly read highly enlarged print. Perhaps this exchange between Nigel and Adrian Mole expresses how she felt about losing her sight:

> Nigel rang to tell me that he is suffering from post-blindness depression. In an attempt to counsel him, I asked him what was the worst thing about being blind.
>
> Nigel snapped, 'I can't fucking see!'[28]

From Luka Kille's drawings to Sue Townsend's books, art can provide a method of explaining visual loss to those of us with good sight. Although anyone can simulate sight loss for a few minutes by closing their eyes, knowing that you can open your eyes at any time and see again avoids the psychological impact of blindness. Having said that, when I asked Luka whether she felt other people should experiment with being blindfolded for several days, her face lit up – of course they should! As she reminisced, she became nostalgic about her eight days without sight:

> It was actually really relaxing because I really noticed everything, every little nuance of what I was doing. I can see at some point in the future this being sold as a retreat. We have silent retreats, maybe we will have sensory deprivation retreats because it just enhances your state of mindfulness and rest.

Notes

1 Trevor-Roper, 1997.
2 Fletcher, Schuchard and Renninger, 2012.
3 Crabb et al., 2013.
4 '5 music videos', 2022.

5   Godin, 2021.
6   Clayton, accessed 31 March 2022.
7   Hawkins, 2014.
8   Living Paintings, 'Our books', accessed 19 April 2022.
9   Living Paintings, 'Trustees' Report', accessed 19 April 2022.
10 Kleege, 2018.
11 Chakraborty, 2018.
12 Sengupta, 2020.
13 Kilcrease, 2016.
14 '99% invisible', 2010.
15 Kleege, 1999.
16 Leland, 2021.
17 Björk, 2000.
18 Bashinky, 2017.
19 Holmström, 1993.
20 Bharwani et al., 2016.
21 Ribowsky, 2010.
22 Lynskey, 2012.
23 Dale, Sakkalou and Osborne, 2021.
24 ABC news, 2017.
25 Fenby, 1966.
26 Townsend, 2012.
27 BBC, 2016.
28 Townsend, 2004.

3
The visible deterrent: employment and education with vision impairment

Piotr's bulky build and dirty work clothes gave me a false impression. Although he looked like a builder, he was an English literature graduate from a top university in Warsaw and being a labourer was a temporary phase.

'All my life they told me I was a blind child – I can't do this and I can't do that,' he explained. 'So I said: "I'll come to London and not tell anyone I can't see, see what happens."' A mischievous grin played across his mouth, beneath his eyes, which beat left to right with nystagmus.

Nystagmus is one of the giveaway signs of vision impairment. Unlike the roving, random eye movements of someone like Stevie Wonder, nystagmus is a regular wobble of the eyes, like a sped-up pendulum. Generally, the eyes drift to one side fairly slowly, then will jump back to the other side, four or five times every second. Most people experience nystagmus sometimes – if you watch someone trying to read a platform name from a moving train, you'll see their eyes follow the sign, then jump back to the next sign which appears. However, Piotr had nystagmus because he had oculocutaneous albinism – a rare condition which affects about one in 17,000 people and is characterised by a lack of pigment in hair, skin and eye cells. This lack of eye pigment causes sensitivity to light and reduced vision. The iris of someone with albinism is usually pale blue, with a reddish-pink tinge. (Brown irises have brown pigment, but people with blue eyes don't have blue pigment in the iris; they appear that colour only due to the wavelengths of light reflected back to the person looking at them). As well as these pigmentary changes, people with albinism have structural differences in the visual system. Their retina does not have a fovea (the 'pit' in the centre of the retina which has the most closely packed cells, usually associated with the best visual acuity and damaged in macular disease) and their optic nerves do not cross in the centre of the brain in the same way as someone without albinism.

Although he was eligible, Piotr declined the offer of being registered as sight impaired, along with its associated benefits, such as a Freedom Pass for free transport around London. Almost defiantly, he worked in a series of jobs where you would think sight is critical. His first job in London was at a bakery. He told me how he lost that job:

> I could bake the bread rolls fine, but they just looked like a blur. It was fine, but one morning the boss caught me touching all the rolls to count them and he shouted at me. As he was shouting he looked at my eyes and said: 'Are you blind?!' I told him 'yes' and walked out. I hated the early mornings anyway.

Piotr's self-confidence is unusual for someone with such a visible sign of poor sight. Teenagers, in particular, can be extremely self-conscious about meeting new people and dating. They think their nystagmus will be the first thing people see and will lead to rejection. Indeed, in a paper surveying the opinions of children with visual impairment, one 12-year-old girl said:

> When I meet boys and look them in the eyes, they see my eyes wobble. That's what might put them off … If there was like a surgery to stop my eyes wobbling, I wouldn't care about my eye problem, it's just the wobbling; that's what affects me the most.[1]

There is an operation which theoretically helps nystagmus, but it is drastic – the tendon around every eye muscle is cut. Even such dramatic surgery tends to give disappointing results. Instead, people with nystagmus devise strategies to divert attention away from their wobbling eyes: a bold haircut or unusual pair of glasses can be the first thing people notice.

Piotr had realised these adaptations aren't always necessary. He had a shaved head and didn't wear glasses but relied on the fact that most people are like his bakery boss and just aren't that observant. He loved living in London and breaking free from the restrictions placed on him as a blind person. He went to the theatre every week, using a small pair of binoculars to make out what was happening on stage. He'd also fallen in love and his clearly devoted girlfriend was sitting in the room with him.

One of the key parts of my job is ensuring people are safe. I will refer someone for mobility training if they can't cross the road, to their local rehabilitation team if they can't cook without burning themselves, or to a falls team if they trip over. So I was naturally concerned when Piotr told me that his next job after the bakery was on a building site, which would surely have endangered him, and probably others.

'Do you think you were safe on the building site?' I asked. The mischievous grin reappeared.

'Oh no,' he said. 'One time I fell through a hole and had to do this' – here he pointed his elbows out, like a child impersonating a chicken – 'and saved myself, otherwise I would have fallen two floors.'

I was struggling to phrase that he might perhaps want to consider a safer job when he reassured me by interrupting:

'But next week I start a new job. I will be a store detective,' he said, proudly.

'And do you think your sight will allow you to do that?' I asked.

At this, he sat upright in the chair, and pronounced: 'I will be a visible deterrent.'

Piotr's story is amusing but unusual. People with vision impairment are twice as likely to be unemployed as those with good sight in countries like the UK, Singapore, Canada and Australia, even if they have higher educational qualifications.[2–5] For those who do have jobs, 'under-employment' is common, where the person would like to work more hours, or in a more demanding job, than they currently are.[2] In lower-income countries, the unemployment rate for people with any type of disability is even higher. Researchers from Ghana say that 'in sub-Saharan Africa, disability is synonymous with poverty, hardship and poor living conditions'.[6]

Blind schools

One reason for the high unemployment rate in blind people who want to work might be the careers advice given to children with poor sight. Journalist Peter White, the longstanding presenter of *In Touch* and *You and Yours* on BBC Radio 4, writes that in the 1960s careers advice for blind people was limited to 'Good with your brain: lawyer. Good with your hands: physiotherapist. Don't want to do either of those: clearly you were a bit of a misfit who would have to sink or swim on your own.'[7] Sadly this does not seem to have improved over the past 50 years, with a 2020 report from the Thomas Pocklington Trust showing inconsistencies in careers advice for young people with vision impairment. Only half of the teenagers they interviewed had met with a careers advisor and only one-third had completed a work experience placement.[8] A teacher for vision impairment interviewed for this report highlighted the risks of young people with sight loss ending up as someone not in education, employment or training (sometimes called 'NEET'):

> Some young people I think have had careers guidance in college that hasn't really hit the spot, so they have left college and ended up NEET on their sofa.[8]

Being involuntarily NEET can be bad for mental health and wellbeing, although some people fill the gaps with volunteering, hobbies and other activities. Having lots of people unavailable for work is also bad for the economy, which is perhaps why blind schools were developed in the Victorian era.

Peter White attended New College Worcester, a residential school established in 1866 as the 'Worcester College for the Blind Sons of Gentlemen' and currently run by the Royal National Institute of Blind People. By 1918 its graduates had become clergymen, teachers, solicitors, masseurs and farmers. In its early years, the criterion for entrance was to be 'too blind to be able to read the ordinary school books used by children'.[9] This quite liberal definition allowed children with reasonably good sight to obtain blind scholar grants, which were in demand as blind schools at that time had high standards, at least for boys. Girls with vision impairment weren't catered for until 1921, when the 'Chorleywood College for Girls with Little or No Sight' opened.[10] In 1987, New College and the Chorleywood College merged to form the current New College Worcester, and the school is now open to boys and girls aged 11 to 19.

Peter White describes the school's annual 'Founder's Day,' 29th May,[11] as a day when all pupils were required to leave the school grounds and were allowed to go wherever they wanted. At the age of 11, Peter went to Dudley Zoo for the day (on a repeat visit, two years later, he also drove a dodgem car). In his final year he spent Founder's Day hitchhiking more than 100 miles to visit his mother for a surprise visit.

The rival 'Royal Normal College and Academy for the Blind' opened in 1872 in South London and provided more vocational education. The name 'normal' came from the French *école normale*, meaning a school which provides advanced tuition in one field, in this case music, as the school aimed to train blind organists, teachers and piano tuners. By 1885 it had 170 pupils using facilities which included two gyms, a swimming pool and two roller-skating rinks. The school still exists as a Further Education college, although it is now called the Royal National College for the Blind, has moved to Hereford and has greatly reduced its roller-skating facilities. Perhaps the most famous alumnus of this college is the former home secretary David Blunkett. A contemporary of Peter White, Blunkett had slightly more productive careers advice, with his advisor finding him a job as a copy typist for the East Midlands Gas Board. A member of the Labour Party all his adult life, Blunkett became a union steward and was elected as Member of Parliament for Sheffield Brightside in 1987.

Blunkett also attended a boarding school for the earlier years of his education – at the Manchester Road School for the Blind in Sheffield. In his memoir *On a Clear Day,* Blunkett describes how the blind children at this school could avoid the 'lights out' rule by reading braille in bed, before they moved on to listening to pirate radio stations as they got a little older. Being at a school for blind children does not seem to have limited his activities. As well as conventional lessons, he recalls sledging, cycling, riding go-karts (not always without crashing into the head-teacher's study window) and letting off fireworks.[12] While at the Royal Normal College, Blunkett chipped one of his front teeth in a boisterous game of jousting (standing on chairs, using rolled-up braille magazines as lances), an injury which is still visible today.

Alongside these blind schools, classes were developed for children with moderate vision impairment who could still access enlarged print. The first class for children with low vision, rather than no vision, was opened in 1908 at Boundary Lane School in Camberwell, London, by Dr James Kerr and ophthalmologist Nathaniel Bishop Harman. Although initially called the 'myope class', Kerr acknowledged that this name was misleading and later suggested that 'sight saving classes' might have been a better title. Some of the first children taught in this class had corneal diseases, inflammatory eye diseases like choroiditis and keratitis, or albinism.[13]

The class adjusted the curriculum in three ways: work which might cause eye strain was limited; physical education excluded exercises which might cause retinal detachment; and there were more manual lessons such as handicraft, model-making, carpentry and drawing.[14] Children went into the mainstream class when learning could be achieved by listening to the teacher, returning to the myope class for lessons involving reading or writing. For physical education drill and dance were encouraged, but football and violent games were prohibited.

Staff received additional instruction in teaching children with vision impairment and the classes were small, with at most 20 students for each teacher. The school quickly developed to use print, not braille. Kerr stated that 'With the root ideas at the start there might at first have been inscribed "books, paper, pencils or pens cannot enter here" … experience has somewhat modified this veto.' This quotation has been taken literally by some; since it first appeared in a 1943 book by Winifred Hathaway,[16] several textbooks have falsely claimed that this phrase was indeed painted over the door.[17]

Children read large print and wrote large letters on blackboards or black linen rollers. Bishop Harman decided that 'We want a library of large printed books, or rather scrolls … printed in letters of such a size that a child with, say, 6/24 vision can read with ease at the distance of two or three metres.'[18]

Reading small print was discouraged. Kerr advised parents 'for the protection of your children's eyes … do not let it (sic) read or write,' and children were told that reading for pleasure was a vice until they were fully grown.[13] To discourage children from reading their own writing, a shield was fixed to pens so that the nib and writing could not be seen, and children were told to look away when writing on the blackboard. In maths, no marks were awarded for long division if it was written down, as Kerr thought 'the purposes of life for the majority can be well met by mental arithmetic'.[13]

The welfare of children with vision impairment was considered carefully. Dr Bishop Harman advocated the inclusion of this class within a mainstream school, recognising the stigma associated with attending a blind school.[14,18] In a chilling precursor of Hitler's Germany, Kerr warned: 'In some (low vision classes) they are badged red-button children, but it is unwise to label any individual as different.'[15]

The myope school concept spread quickly. By 1913, France and Germany had similar classes and the 'conservation of vision class' was approved by the Boston Board of Education in the USA, following a visit to London by Edward Allen of the Perkins Institution for the Blind. In 1915 there were myope classes in Birmingham, Brighton, Bristol, Bolton, Exeter, Leicester, Leeds, Liverpool, Nottingham, Oldham, Sheffield and Stoke-on-Trent.[19]

Substitute 'the written word' for 'iPads and smartphones' and many of Kerr's recommendations sound surprisingly contemporary. Nearly a century ago he was concerned by 'the young student … using the eyes in an intensive way, far beyond what any generations before have done'. He also advocated time outdoors. Parents of myopic children were advised to 'get the little one interested in games and outside play', advice which is now known to limit the development of myopia.[20] In the 1910s, myope classrooms deliberately had large amounts of natural light; today, China is experimenting with glass classrooms to limit myopia progression.[21]

The Boundary Lane School no longer exists (like many public buildings in London, it has been converted to private apartments) and most children with vision impairment are educated alongside children with good vision in mainstream schools, sometimes being taken out of the class for additional lessons in braille or mobility. Some children will have the help of a one-to-one learning support assistant, but increasingly technology can be used to help them access the curriculum. Whiteboard content is relayed wirelessly to a screen on the student's desk and electronic textbooks are shown in enlarged high-contrast print, presented on a braille display or read aloud over headphones.

Tactile teaching aids are used in all sorts of lessons. A blind child might handle a 3D printed model of a brain in biology, an embossed painting in art, then a tactile astronomical map in physics. The Tactile Universe project at the University of Portsmouth provides open source 3D printer files for accurate models of galaxies, under the direction of vision-impaired astrophysicist Dr Nic Bonne. Bonne avoided the limited careers advice which was provided to Peter White and was not deterred from working in astrophysics. He writes: 'Sometimes it surprises me that nobody has ever said to me "But you're blind! Why did you choose astronomy as a job?" I hope that if they had, it wouldn't have changed my mind. To be honest, it might have made me doubt myself though.'[22]

Vision impairment in the workplace

The United Nations Convention on the Rights of Persons with Disabilities, signed by 164 countries, recognises the rights of people with disability to work on an equal basis with others.[23] In the UK, the Equality Act 2010 identifies disability as a protected characteristic, meaning that reasonable adjustments must be made to allow someone with vision impairment to work. These adjustments might include providing a larger monitor, improving office lighting or providing additional software so an employee can dictate their correspondence rather than typing it, for example. What exactly constitutes 'reasonable adjustment' is not well defined. It is clearly reasonable for a bank clerk with vision impairment to have a larger monitor so they can see the screen more easily, but it would be ridiculous for a blind bus driver to be employed with an assistant to drive the bus for them.

Other countries have adopted these principles in slightly different ways. In Canada, employers have a 'duty to accommodate';[24] in India, 1 per cent of government jobs are reserved for people with vision impairment, hearing loss or locomotor disability;[25] and Japan's Disabled Persons' Fundamental Law allows the government to 'collect levies from employers who fail to employ the required number of persons with disabilities', with the money being given to employers who employ more disabled people.[26]

When recruiting new workers, employers must provide application forms in accessible formats and adapt any interview tests to make them easier to see.[27] I am often asked whether people with vision impairment should declare their sight loss on their application form, at an interview or once they have been offered the job, but I don't have a good answer for this. It is very difficult to prove that someone hasn't been offered a job because they declared a disability on their application, but would someone with vision impairment want to work for an employer who doesn't engage with their sight loss during the recruitment process? Even children are aware of this. In the research, which surveyed the views of young people with sight loss, a 15-year-old boy said:

> If, say, there's a job going round and I've got an eyesight problem and someone else hasn't, then they'll probably pick the person who hasn't got the eyesight problem, because they will be easier to employ.[1]

Although this boy identifies the additional difficulty that people with vision impairment experience in finding work, most young adults I meet in the low vision clinic are in employment, or are comfortable with not working. As an example, in the last two months in the low vision clinic I have met a teacher, a civil servant, two shop workers, a bookkeeper for a small business, a taxi dispatcher, a hospital play specialist, a statistician, a postal worker, two academics, a publican and a nurse. Some of these people had received a formal workplace assessment and had assistive technology provided, but most had come to an arrangement with their employer where they requested the extra help they needed. In some cases, this was a larger monitor or extra lighting; in other cases it was having different duties (extra classroom sessions in exchange for not having to watch children in the playground at break) or adaptations in the workplace (the nurse received notes from the doctor in her practice in thick black pen, rather than thin blue fountain pen she used to use). Over my career, I have met people with occupations which might be considered surprising for someone with vision impairment, including animators, video editors and television reviewers. A common factor in their workplace happiness seems to be the quality and understanding of their immediate boss – something which is probably true for every employee, sight impaired or not.

Visual standards for workplaces

Reasonable adjustments can be made for many professions, but some occupations have legal vision standards which prohibit people with vision impairment from performing that work. Driving is the most frequent example. Lorry drivers, pilots and bus drivers have more stringent vision requirements than car drivers. Strict standards exist for pilots, firefighters, electricians and railway workers, who must also have good colour vision. Police officers and prison guards need to have a minimum standard of vision without glasses, in case their spectacles are damaged or knocked off in a fight.

Some professions have less formal vision requirements, allowing the person to self-certify that they are able to perform the job. For example, medical doctors in the UK have to declare whether they have a health condition which may affect the clinical care they provide, which is then assessed on a case-by-case basis.[28]

There is a precedent for a blind person becoming a doctor. Despite being blind from birth and being the seventh child in a poor migrant family, Jacob Bolotin was admitted to Chicago Medical School and graduated in 1912. After qualification he became an expert in heart and lung disease and a sought-after speaker. In one of his speeches, he elegantly demonstrated the principle of reasonable adjustment:

> Well, is there anything so remarkable about it? Because a man has no eyes, is it any sign that he hasn't any brains? That is the trouble with the world and the blind man. All the blind man asks is fair play. Give him an equal chance without prejudice, and he generally manages to hold his own with his more fortunate colleagues.[29]

It is more common for doctors to lose their sight after qualification, as happened to Thomas Rhodes Armitage. Born in 1824, Armitage studied at King's College London and became a physician based in London's affluent Marylebone district. After vision impairment forced him to retire from medical practice, he led the 'Indigent Blind Visiting Society', the forerunner to the Royal National Institute of Blind People. He also donated nearly £40,000 to the Royal Normal College. He lived a full life, with his obituary in the *British Medical Journal* reporting that he died 'following serious injuries sustained by his horse falling and rolling over him', at the age of 66.[30]

In most countries doctors do not have to pass a colour vision test, even though colour coding is used throughout hospitals, for differentiating between different blood tubes, different anaesthetic drugs or different gauges of needles. As ophthalmologist and colour vision researcher Peter Thomas says, 'Many doctors will know that a purple blood tube is used to collect specimens for erythrocyte sedimentation rate. Fewer would know to seek out a tube containing ethylenediaminetetraacetic acid to perform the same test.'[31] Although colour coding can still be useful for people without good colour vision, the colours should be suitably different to ensure they can be easily recognised. About one in 20 men will be unable to differentiate between red and green, for example, but far fewer will confuse purple and orange. It is good practice to use other markers alongside colour coding, such as different patterns. An example of this is the colour-blind version of the London Underground map, where lines are identified by different patterns rather than the colours used on the regular map.[32] This can even be seen by people with achromatopsia, an extremely rare condition where people do not see colour at all.

Blind sport

For visually impaired sportspeople, there are maximum standards of vision determined by the International Blind Sports Federation and used by the International Paralympic Committee. Assessing a professional athlete with a vision impairment is probably the only time when I meet people who are disappointed that their vision isn't poorer.

These criteria vary by sport, but in general B1 is used for people with 'no useful sight', sometimes called 'totals' by people in the blind sport community. B2 includes people with visual acuity up to about 1/60 (that is, about 60 times poorer than 'perfect' sight) or with a very severely constricted visual field of less than 10 degrees. People whose vision is better than this but who still fall into the World Health Organization's definition of 'severe vision impairment' (see Table 1.1) are classified as B3.[33] Some organisations also have categories of B4 and B5 for people with better levels of vision, but these are not used in international competitions.

Some sports require each team to have a mix of people with different levels of vision impairment. For example, a blind cricket team must have at least four players who are classified as B1, three players who are B2 and up to three B3 players. In other sports, such as blind football, all the players (except the goalkeeper) are blindfolded to equalise the vision between each participant. David Blunkett writes about the joy of football for someone with vision impairment coming from the '50 per cent of the time we connected with the ball rather than thin air or someone's shins'.[12]

Another sport where everyone is blindfolded is goalball, which allows people with good sight to play the sport alongside people with vision impairment. I have been invited to play goalball a few times but have never been brave enough to try. In this sport, each team of three players tries to get a large, heavy, bell-filled ball past the opposing team, throwing it at speeds of up to 60 kilometres per hour. It's an exciting sport to watch, although spectators have to remain silent during play.

Different sports have different modifications for athletes with vision impairment. Some cyclists and runners have sighted guides who ride or run alongside them, blind football and cricket use balls which make a noise, while in visually impaired judo the participants start by touching each other rather than standing apart, as in conventional judo.

Vision impairment caused by the workplace

Eye injuries were a common side effect of working in manual jobs, particularly before the introduction of the Health and Safety at Work Act in 1974. A textbook on eye injuries from the 1940s has examples of posters which would have been displayed in the workplace before the onus of avoiding injuries was placed on employers rather than workers. These posters are often striking, such as the red and black image of a sad face, wearing an eyepatch, surrounded by the slogan 'I didn't … protect my eyes' (Figure 3.1), or the phrase 'He didn't use eye protection. Do you?' beneath a cartoon picture of a man with dark glasses and a white cane. Many of these were created by the artist Hans Arnold Rothholz. Despite being born in Germany and being detained as an 'enemy alien' in the UK during the Second World War, he created a series of British wartime public information posters, publicising war bonds and encouraging people to avoid making long telephone calls. In peacetime he turned his talents to work for the post office ('Post early for Christmas'; 'Is your wireless licensed?'), for London Transport ('Signs that signify

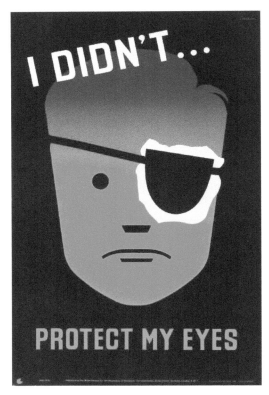

Figure 3.1 A man wearing a patch over his left eye, as a result of not wearing protective goggles. Colour lithograph after L. Cusden, commissioned by the Royal Society for Prevention of Accidents advising employees to wear eye protection. Attribution 4.0 International (CC BY 4.0). Source: Wellcome Collection.

service') and the Royal Society for the Prevention of Accidents ('Here lies the victim of an untied shoelace'). The same textbook breaks down eye injuries by object (80 per cent flying objects, 2.5 per cent explosions) and by industry (the metal and machinery sectors were particularly dangerous).[34]

Today, most eye injuries I see are from leisure activities rather than work. Squash balls are the same size as the eye, so a direct hit damages the eye far more than a tennis ball, where the impact is absorbed by the orbital bones around the eye. Bank holiday weekends bring a rush of people into eye casualty with injuries from DIY, whereas gardening injuries tend to present a few days later, when a fungal infection might have taken hold. Eye protection is important in the home, particularly for the 2 per cent or so of the population who have amblyopia (a 'lazy' eye) and already don't see well from one eye. Eye injuries are far more significant if you don't have another eye to compensate for any vision loss, making the lifetime risk of blindness higher in people with amblyopia.[35]

Miners' nystagmus

Unpleasant workplaces don't only increase the risk of sight loss from injury. In the 1890s, doctors in mining villages across Europe started seeing coalminers who complained of severe, constant headaches, giddiness and being disoriented. Their eyes were bloodshot, sensitive to light and had unusual movements – in some cases, the eyelids would spasm uncontrollably, while others had nystagmus, like Piotr.

How could nystagmus, often associated with severe vision impairment, be caused by coal mining? It is thought to be connected to the extreme darkness of the workplace. As children would have started mining at about eight years of age and would spend six or seven days per week underground, it is not an exaggeration to describe their life as being similar to having vision impairment. In a 1913 lecture, Dr Lister Llewellyn described 700 young men with miners' nystagmus, with an average of 26 years 'of underground life' each.[36] He found the mean light level at their place of work to be 0.018 footcandles – darker than a moonlit night, and 500 times dimmer than the gloomiest tube station platform today. By this time, doctors in the mining district of Liège had already found that the incidence of nystagmus went down with brighter mine lighting, but Davy lamps, life-saving in coal mines, couldn't be made bright enough.

Some doctors remained sceptical about miners' nystagmus, pointing out that about one in 20 people can make their eyes shake voluntarily. These doctors assumed miners' nystagmus was a deliberate ruse to avoid working in the mine. Despite the atrocious working conditions in British coal mines, there was relatively good support for injured and sickened miners, with generous payments made to people suffering from any disease related to their work. Miners' nystagmus was classified as a work-related disease in 1906, then in 1913 the features of the condition were extended to include more subjective characteristics (such as aversion to bright light), arguably making it easier to simulate.[37] By 1938, 1.4 per cent of miners were medically retired through miners' nystagmus. Nystagmus 'deniers' point out that the disease was virtually unheard of in the USA, where mining conditions were similar but where people with occupational diseases did not receive compensation.[38] More evidence for the 'putting it on' hypothesis comes from epidemiology. The first cases were clustered in one colliery in Derbyshire, before spreading through the East Midlands and across the country. This would make sense for an infectious disease, but the 'pseudo-disease' advocates say that this reflects word-of-mouth transmission of a way to escape work: an early example of the odious 'benefit scroungers' narrative perpetuated by today's right-wing press.

New reports of miners' nystagmus petered out in the 1940s, by which time electric light was being used in coal mines, but throughout the twentieth century similar diseases were seen in other occupational groups including soldiers, Genoan crane operators and American railroad dispatchers. More recently, neurologists reported a case of nystagmus in a woman with severe migraine, who lived almost entirely in darkness to alleviate her headaches.[39]

Parenting with vision impairment

It would be naïve to write about work without considering the huge amount of unpaid care work that is done, usually by women, in looking after children, family members with disability or older relatives.

Early in my career, I was shocked to meet someone who didn't want to get her eyes tested as she was convinced she was going blind (she wasn't) and she thought she would have her daughter taken into care if she lost her sight (she wouldn't). This person was wrong to think that vision impairment would lead to her losing the care of her child in the UK in the 1990s, unless she was neglectful or abusive for unconnected reasons, but there is a horribly recent history of blind people being told they shouldn't have children. Gaylen Kapperman, Professor Emeritus at Northern Illinois University, describes a routine visit to his ophthalmologist in the mid-twentieth century:

> He asked me if I had a girlfriend. I said yes, I did. He then asked if I planned to marry her. At that time, marriage had not been uppermost in my mind. I thought about it for a moment and said, yes perhaps! He said, well, then you need to have a vasectomy.[40]

Kapperman ignored this advice, literally running from the doctor's office and jumping in a taxi. He continues: 'As I write this, I have one very wonderful daughter who actually is my genetic daughter and has some of my characteristics – something I would not have, had I obeyed the doctor's orders.'[40]

The theologian and academic John Hull describes his experiences as a blind parent in his diaries, which were published in 1990 as the book *Touching the Rock*. By the time his son is three years old, he understands that "'Show Daddy" means "put whatever you've got in your hand into my hand and you will get it straight back."' Even at the age of two, Thomas Hull knew his father perceived the world differently: 'Pointing to one of his own books, he remarked "Daddy can't read this" and then, pointing to the braille label in a picture book, "Thomas can't read that."' John Hull's wife sometimes needed to remind him to put the lights on when he was in a dark room with his children, leading him to speculate that Thomas grew up thinking his dad could see in the dark, navigating equally well with and without lights on.[41]

The child of a blind parent will sometimes become more independent at an earlier stage. I often meet people in the clinic whose response to the question 'How do you read bills and correspondence?' is 'Oh, my son reads it to me,' even when that child is of primary school age.

Lucia Carver described the experience of living with a blind parent as her supplemental essay for admission to university in the USA. Her father, Kelly, converted a decrepit fraternity house into a wonderfully welcoming guest house for academics visiting the University of Minnesota, which was so popular that when he retired and closed the business it merited a story in the *Minnesota Daily* newspaper.[42] I stayed there several times when performing postdoctoral research with Gordon Legge and it was a special place; I was quoted in the newspaper article as saying that guests could 'have breakfast with a transplant surgeon from Chile, make dinner and chat [with] a Japanese postdoctoral student or play chess with maybe an Egyptian psychologist'. I have fond memories of many happy meals in Kelly's kitchen, extending well into the evening, while the Minnesotan snow piled up outside.

Lucia's essay starts with an anecdote: 'So a blind man is walking along Navy Pier and crashes into a woman in a wheelchair … Sounds like the opening line of a bad joke, doesn't it? If only it was, and not what actually happened to my father during our trip to Chicago,' and ends with a reflection on how her father's vision impairment has made her more stoic, writing that 'my dad has taught me the importance of accepting the things beyond our control. He has accepted his blindness and the possibility he may one day lose all remaining sight.' She closes by almost daring the college authorities to reject her application: 'If he can not only come to terms with such a daunting possibility, but thrive despite it, then there is no reason I can't deal with much less serious problems, like a bad hair day or a college rejection letter.' This bold strategy worked, as Lucia was accepted into both Harvard and Yale.

Blindisms

Although Piotr's boss in the bakery didn't notice it, nystagmus is a fairly obvious sign of vision impairment. Other visible 'blindisms' that some people with severe sight loss display include roving eye movements, eye poking, head movement, staring at lights and body rocking. These signs can appear similar to the mannerisms displayed by some people with autism and are thought to perhaps be a way of self-stimulation for children who have less sensory experience of the world. Eye poking, in particular, can generate phosphenes – flashes of light – even in people with very severe vision impairment.

In her paper comparing children in Nigeria and England, Theresa Abang has shown that body rocking is more common in blind children in the UK, with those in Nigeria being more likely to roll their eyes instead. She attributes this to the lower amount of physical contact between children and their parents in European societies. In particular she highlights the fact that babies in Nigeria are usually carried on their mother's back, limiting the chance of sensory deprivation.[43]

Blindisms are perceived as negative by many people in society, can make employment difficult and can be harmful. Eye poking can cause significant injury, as can rigorous head shaking. Several treatments to overcome these repetitive behaviours have been tried, including punishment (shouting 'no'), blocking the behaviour (holding the child's hand for a few seconds) and reinforcing positive behaviour by giving toys or food. A combination of reinforcement along with brief periods of restraint appears to be the most effective strategy, although evidence for any of these interventions is limited.[44]

Music therapy has also shown promise in reducing blindisms, particularly body rocking. Encouraging children to move their body in time with music allows them to modify their behaviour and to pay more attention to their other senses. Music therapy groups promote sociali-sation and interaction between children; for example, by passing an instrument around the group and by taking turns in playing music.[45]

The persecution of people with albinism

Having pale skin and blond hair wasn't a big problem for Piotr growing up in Poland, but it can have dramatic consequences for children in parts of the world where white skin is unusual. The birth of a child with white skin and hair would cause surprise in many rural African communities, but in some regions those with albinism are persecuted or even killed. In parts of the African Great Lakes region, particularly Malawi and Tanzania, body parts of people with albinism are used in traditional medicine. In other parts of sub-Saharan Africa, there is a false belief that sexual activity with someone with albinism can cure HIV/AIDS.[46] A woman with albinism from Nigeria was blamed for an upsurge in deaths of men within her community and escaped to France, where she was granted asylum. The charity Under the Same Sun educates communities across the world about albinism and has produced a film called *White and Black: Crimes of Colour* which is shown across Tanzania.[47]

Even in a diverse city like London, it is difficult for children to grow up with their appearance not matching their ethnicity. A few years ago, I met Abdullah in the low vision clinic. He was struggling as a Somalian child who didn't look like his peers – people were often surprised to see him at the mosque or speaking Somali. At school he felt that he didn't quite fit in to the Somalian, Muslim or White European community; he told me that he felt outside every group. I referred Abdullah to a counsellor and suggested he may want to join the Albinism Fellowship, a charity that offers support and social activities for children with albinism from all over the world.

Today, Abdullah is able to talk about his condition in a more light-hearted way. For example, he made me laugh when he told me that he was the first person in his entire family to need sun cream in the UK. When I last saw him in the clinic, I showed Abdullah a telescope to use on trips to the theatre with his GCSE drama group. I pointed out that this might make him look a bit different to everyone else in his class, but would enable him to see the stage more easily. He gave me a cheeky grin, pushed his hand through his curly blond hair and said 'To be honest, mate, I don't think it's the telescope that makes me look different.'

Notes

1 Tadić et al., 2015.
2 McCarty, Burgess and Keeffe, 1999.

3 Shaw, Gold and Wolffe, 2007.
4 Cumberland and Rahi, 2016.
5 Chai et al., 2021.
6 Odame et al., 2021.
7 White, 1999.
8 Hewett and Brydon, 2020.
9 Elementary Education Act, 1893.
10 Pritchard, 1963.
11 White, 2021.
12 Blunkett and MacCormick, 2002.
13 Kerr, 1925.
14 House of Commons Board of Education, 1919.
15 Kerr, 1925.
16 Hathaway, 1943.
17 Corn and Erin, 2010.
18 Harman, 1913.
19 Harman, 1915.
20 Rose, 2008.
21 Zhou et al., 2017.
22 Bonne, 2018.
23 United Nations, 2006.
24 CNIB, 2019.
25 DREDF, 2016.
26 WeCapable, accessed 22 June 2022.
27 RNIB, accessed 22 June 2022.
28 General Medical Council, accessed 22 June 2022.
29 Kendrick, 2008.
30 'Thomas Rhodes Armitage', 1890.
31 Thomas et al., 2021.
32 Transport for London, 2002.
33 International Blind Sports Federation, accessed 2022.
34 Minton, 1949.
35 Rahi et al., 2002.
36 Llewellyn, 1913.
37 Davis, 2001.
38 Fishman, 2006.
39 Kamourieh et al., 2021.
40 Kapperman, 2019.
41 Hull, 1990.
42 Anderson, 2019.
43 Abang, 1985.
44 Ivy and Ledford, 2022.
45 Gourgey, 1998.
46 Nkrumah, 2019.
47 Under the Same Sun, accessed 7 June 2022.

4
Supernoses and birdlistening: other senses in vision impairment

Muriel has a supernose. Three times a week, she takes a train from North London to an industrial estate near Heathrow Airport, where she helps to develop some of the world's most exclusive and expensive perfumes.

As soon as Muriel told me her about her superpower, I moved my chair backwards slightly. I was horrified to imagine what she would be able to tell from my odour, immediately imagining her as an olfactory Sherlock Holmes: 'You cycled to work this morning; your bike chain is too oily and some of it is on your right trouser leg; you were running late and sweated when passing a diesel-powered bus; you use Original Source shower gel, and last had a bath on … Tuesday?'

The evolutionary reason for humans having a sense of smell is unclear. It's known to play a role in mate selection and might be used by infants to recognise family members and differentiate them from strangers. Strong smells can warn of danger, which is perhaps why sniffing a milk bottle after opening it is almost a reflex action for many people. Pregnant women often have a heightened sense of smell, to protect the unborn child from maternal food poisoning. Some doctors believe this heightened sense of smell is a cause of the inaccurately named 'morning' sickness.

Muriel only noticed her sense of smell was so good when she became severely sight impaired. As someone with retinitis pigmentosa, her vision had been deteriorating since her teens. Little by little, her visual field shrank to encompass an area of about five degrees, so when she looked at someone's nose she couldn't tell if they were wearing a hat or not. Her vision was too poor to drive, she relied on a white cane to walk safely, and her cat had a sadistic habit of tripping her over.

Muriel explained to me how she realised her sense of smell was so good. 'When I was on the street I could smell when people were close to me. It was often the only way I knew someone was about to walk past: I'd catch a whiff of their perfume, or their body odour, before I'd see them or even hear them.' When she heard a radio programme about 'super-smellers' she contacted a perfumier directly.

The selection process was tough. Using the brilliantly named 'Sniffin' Sticks' test, Muriel had to identify which of three sticks smelt different to the other two. The intensity of the smell reduced until most people wouldn't be able to perceive anything at all, but Muriel kept passing the tests. This confirmed her status as someone with hyperosmia – a heightened sense of smell.

Hyperosmia isn't necessarily a good thing – I'm sure it's a blessing not to be able to smell communal rubbish bins a hundred metres away, and Muriel mentioned that public transport could be difficult. 'People put on *so* much perfume!' she told me. 'It's like they've had a bath in it! Just one dab, that's all anyone needs. If I'm on the train and everyone has perfume on, it's just awful!'

Is Muriel's sense of smell any better because of her vision impairment? Some people who have been blind from birth have changes in the structure of their brain that may give an advantage to the sense of smell. Studies have shown a larger olfactory bulb (part of the forebrain associated with smell)[1] and that the visual cortex in some blind people responds to smelly stimuli,[2,3] which may theoretically be associated with a better ability to detect smells. However, larger studies of people with acquired blindness, like Muriel, have not shown any improvements in odour discrimination (the ability to identify a specific smell) or olfactory threshold (the ability to smell a faint odour)[4] and a meta-analysis of 18 studies has shown no significant differences in either of these skills.[5] It seems most likely that Muriel has always had a very acute sense of smell, but that she has only noticed it more since her vision started to decline.

As well as providing her with an interesting job, Muriel might appreciate another, surprising, benefit from being able to smell so well. A 2018 study showed that people with hyperosmia report more sexual satisfaction than people with normal or reduced smell. The researchers speculated that 'certain body odours may contribute to the concept of sexual pleasure by enhanced recruitment of reward areas'.[6]

The idea of blind people having improvements in their other senses appeals to our sense of fairness, so that losing one sense improves another way of perceiving the world. This belief is common across cultures and is shared by blind people. In 2022, Michal Pieniak and colleagues asked over a hundred people with sight loss to rate their own sense of smell, hearing, touch and taste in comparison to people with perfect sight. They found that people with vision impairment rated their own ability in these senses as better than people with good sight. All of the participants in the study, blind and sighted, also agreed with the general statement: 'In comparison to sighted people, blind people's sense of smell/hearing/taste/touch is [better].'[7] The researchers suggest this is related to a 'conviction that the world is a just place.' However, they also point out that there is very little relationship between people's perceived ability at smelling and objective tests like the Sniffin' Sticks. In other words, people are very bad at knowing how good their sense of smell actually is.

Do blind people hear better?

My friend and colleague Gordon Legge is Professor of Psychology at the University of Minnesota and leads the Minnesota Laboratory for Low Vision Research. He is an international expert in psychophysics, the branch of science that quantifies the brain's response to sensory information, and has a particular interest in how people with vision impairment read print.

Gordon had good sight until he was six years old, when he developed Stevens-Johnson syndrome, a very rare, very serious inflammatory condition. This caused the cornea in both of his eyes to become opaque. Even with strong glasses Gordon has significant vision impairment, with severely reduced visual acuity and contrast sensitivity. At work he uses a combination of technology and human assistance to access the information he needs. A rite of passage for any junior scientist in Gordon's lab is to accompany him to a scientific conference. As Gordon makes braille notes on the spoken content of the presentations, he will ask his student to describe the graphs and images displayed on the slides. I helped with this when I was a visiting postdoctoral scientist in Gordon's lab, sitting next to him as he whispered questions like: 'What do you think, Michael, is that correlation convincing?'

As well as teaching me a huge amount about science, Gordon encouraged me to appreciate baseball, which is one of his passions. As a cricket fan, I am very comfortable with sports that include statistics, long drawn-out matches and detailed radio commentary. On our many visits to watch the Minnesota Twins, I was fascinated by how accurately Gordon could point to action on the field, usually before I'd noticed it, purely on the basis of what he had heard on his portable radio. He has an impressive ability to keep up with the game, listen to the commentary and simultaneously keep up a conversation, peppered with my very basic questions about baseball.

Another of Gordon's hobbies is ornithology. Most birdwatchers use binoculars, but he 'birdlistens' instead. He can identify dozens of birds by their song and is quicker to locate birds than many sighted birdwatchers, especially when the bird is hidden or hard to see.

Does Gordon's ability to listen to the radio commentary and my conversation at the same time reflect the fact that he is better at hearing because of his vision loss, or is it just a reflection of his intelligence? Is he better at localising birds because of an improved auditory system, or has he just honed this skill? The idea that blind people hear better than people with perfect sight is very longstanding and is perhaps the most common trope associated with vision loss.

Gordon's ability to locate objects from their sound is a skill called auditory localisation. For people with vision impairment this is vital, as without good vision it can be lifesaving to be able to hear the position of a bicycle or a car accurately. Several studies have shown that blind people are better at auditory localisation, both in terms of the direction a sound is coming from and how far away it is,[8–10] and that they are better at detecting the movement of a sound.[11] These skills are enhanced in people who lose their vision as adults, as well as those who go blind in childhood, suggesting they are learned. However, people who are blind from birth do not seem to be better at auditory localisation, perhaps as some vision in early childhood can help people learn spatial awareness.[12,13]

As well as being able to locate the source of a sound, people who are blind from childhood are sometimes better at identifying and remembering the pitch of a musical note, although this effect is not seen in people who lose their vision as adults.[14] Musicians who are blind from birth are more likely to have 'perfect pitch' than musicians with good sight.[15]

I am diligent about introducing myself to people with vision impairment every time I meet them. I will always say 'Hi Gordon, it's Michael' rather than just 'Hi Gordon.' This is taught on vision impairment awareness courses and compensates for the fact that blind people can't rely on the visual cues that people with good sight use to recognise someone. However, there is some evidence that blind people are more skilled at recognising voices and linking someone's voice to their name.[16] One study has even shown that the brains of blind people can process sounds more quickly than those with good sight.[17]

The only aspect of hearing that doesn't seem to be improved in blind people is the ability to hear quiet sounds better than anyone else. Even though blind people don't have this superpower, science does support the popular perception that their hearing is better in other ways. Gordon says that he feels people with vision impairment are more attentive to sound, noticing things that go unnoticed by those with better vision.

Touch sensitivity in blind people

Gordon used to subscribe to the braille version of the *New York Times* and uses braille notetaking devices. His desk is piled high with braille paperwork. He clearly has very good touch sensitivity, but is this related to his blindness or just because he has so much practice at reading with his fingertips?

Touch sensitivity is measured in a similar way to visual acuity, where the smallest feature that can be detected is recorded as the 'tactile acuity'. Tactile acuity does seem to be better in blind people than those with good sight.[18] This improvement is similar in people who are blind from birth and those who go blind as adults[19] and does seem to be related to experience, as people with good vision can improve their touch sensitivity with practice[20] and people who use their sense of touch a lot, like pianists, also have better tactile acuity.[21] Pianists and braille users also seem to be resistant to the age-related decline in touch sensitivity that occurs in people who don't spend so much time concentrating on the sensation in their fingertips.[22]

Is this better touch sensitivity due to changes in the brain, or just due to practice? As the chair of one of the world's leading psychology departments (the workplace of the famous B. F. Skinner and others), Gordon is ideally placed to answer this question.

Cross-modal plasticity

Cross-modal plasticity is the term given to the effect when neurons in one region of the brain respond to input from another sense following the loss of sensory input.[23] For example, cross-modal plasticity in a blind person would mean that the visual cortex responds to sound or touch. Our understanding of cross-modal plasticity has improved with each new development in brain scanning, from positron emission tomography

(PET scans) in the 1980s to functional magnetic resonance imaging (fMRI) in the 2000s.

It has been known for decades that the visual cortex in people who are completely blind is still active and that it can respond to touch stimuli: for example, when someone reads braille. What hasn't always been clear is whether this activation is due to mental imagery. Do the cells in the visual cortex respond directly to the sensation in the fingertips of reading braille, or does the visual cortex create a mental image of the shape which the fingers detect?

Gordon reads large print and braille at similar speeds (around a hundred words per minute). Together with his PhD student Sing-Hang Cheung and some colleagues, Gordon devised an experiment to compare what happened in his brain when he read large print and when he read braille.

When Gordon read large print, most of the visual areas of his brain showed increased activity, as expected. However, one region was quiet: the very tip of the occipital cortex, the part of the brain most associated with central vision. In people with good sight, this area responds when they are reading or performing a visually demanding task requiring excellent visual acuity. Gordon's central vision is still intact, although his visual acuity is very reduced in this area. As he writes in their paper: 'Since [Gordon] had no central-visual-field loss, the lack of activity in the foveal confluence is surprising.'[24]

Next, the team looked at what happened when he read braille. This time, the occipital tip was active. Remarkably, in the absence of being able to help Gordon see, the most important visual part of his brain had adapted to process touch.

To answer the question on whether Gordon was visualising the braille symbols when he touched them, he went back into the brain scanner and just imagined the braille characters as symbols. Once again, the occipital tip was quiet, showing that this area only responded to Gordon reading braille characters by touching them.

Finally, two people with good vision had the same scans performed. As they did not read braille, they were asked to count the number of dots they could feel instead. In each case, their visual cortex remained silent when they performed the dot-counting task, showing no braille activation of the visual cortex.

The experiments showed that Gordon did show cross-modal plasticity. In their paper, published in *Current Biology*, the team called this 'experience-dependent cortical reorganisation', writing that 'eventually, the neurons normally adept at resolving visual details were recruited for fine discrimination of tactile details. The rest of the visual neurons continued to process coarse visual information.'[24] I find this astonishing. The part of Gordon's brain devoted to high-acuity vision – indeed the part of his brain that he used for vision for the first six years of his life – now responds to his fingertips instead of his eyes.

As Gordon's brain has adjusted to his blindness, what would happen if he received a new treatment which would restore his eyes to perfect working order? Would it adjust back again, or would this foveal region of his brain still only respond to touch? To answer this question, it is useful to look at the experiences of deaf people who have had their hearing restored with a cochlear implant.

In some deaf people auditory areas of the brain respond to visual input, particularly for seeing sign language.[25] Some clinicians suggest that deaf children waiting for a cochlear implant shouldn't use sign language, as this might create brain plasticity which could limit their hearing after the operation.[26] Less is known about what happens when vision is restored, perhaps as there are fewer cases of people having dramatic improvements in their vision after a long period of blindness, but this study does seem to suggest that, even if Gordon's eyes were miraculously cured, he would still not see as well as someone who has had perfect eyesight for their whole life.[26] Chapter 8 examines sight restoration in more detail.

Braille

Like several braille readers I know, Gordon has visited the town of Coupvray in northern France, Louis Braille's childhood home. Louis Braille had good sight until he was three years old, when an injury in his father's leather workshop damaged one of his eyes (whether it was the right or the left remains unclear). His other eye developed sympathetic ophthalmia, a rare auto-immune response to the injury in his first eye, leaving him with no light perception in either eye by the age of five. At 10, he went to the residential Royal Institute for Blind Youth in Paris.

Tactile writing systems were already in use at the Institute for Blind Youth. Valentin Haüy, the school's founder, provided embossed books, where the letters printed on the page were raised so their shape could be felt with a fingertip. This is a cumbersome and slow way to read, particularly for someone who hasn't already learned to read the printed alphabet before losing their sight.

The idea of encoding letters with raised dots is generally attributed to Charles Barbier de la Serre, an eighteenth-century French artillery officer. After moving to the USA during the French Revolution, Barbier became fascinated by different writing systems, such as those used by native Americans. He developed a 'night writing' system with up to twelve raised dots representing each syllable, so that soldiers could read at night without using lights that might alert the enemy.[27]

Louis Braille was introduced to this writing system when he was 12 years old and Barbier demonstrated his system at the school. According to Braille's biography, he 'indicated several improvements to M. Barbier', and modified the system towards braille as it is known today.[28] Braille's main modifications were to reduce the size of the grid for each letter (from a grid of 2×6 dots to 2×3, so they are less tall and can be felt more quickly), to encode letters rather than syllables and to add punctuation marks, numbers and symbols. Later he developed a system for braille music, combining the pitch with the note duration in a single symbol.

Braille is not a language, but a way of encoding letters in the reader's native tongue. A German person can't read Hungarian braille, but an Australian woman can read the braille *Washington Post*. In standard, uncontracted braille, each symbol represents one letter or punctuation mark, so UCL is written as ∴ ⠉ ⠓, for example.

In Grade 2 or contracted braille, abbreviations are added and some redundant letters are removed. For example, rather than having six letters, 'enough' is written with just one symbol for the letter pair ('en') and 'yourselves' is written with the letters 'yrvs', a little like how my daughter writes text messages. Gordon told me that when his wife Wendy (who has good sight) learned braille, soon after meeting him, she started using these contractions in her written notes, decades before they became fashionable.

Learning braille

The best way to learn braille depends on the age of the person with sight loss. Children who are blind from birth will learn braille at the same stage as their peers learn to read visually, with contracted braille symbols being introduced as they occur naturally in text. Older children who can already read visually are taught braille using a code-based approach, translating the dots into visualised print, before developing the skill to read without making this mental transcription.[29]

For very young children, pre-braille skills like dot counting and manipulation are taught first, before moving on to formal braille symbols. Braille LEGO blocks can be used to teach these skills, as well as when teaching braille itself. In one challenge, children are asked to build sandwiches, putting a block marked 'cheese' in between two bricks embossed with the braille for 'bread'.

It is a common misconception that adults can't be taught braille. I have met many parents of blind children who have learnt braille alongside their children and several older adults who decided to learn this skill later in life, although few are proficient enough to read braille for pleasure. Teachers of vision impairment also learn some braille as part of their training, although they usually need to be blindfolded to avoid the temptation to look at the position of the dots.

About one in every 15 blind people in the UK can read braille,[30] but only half this number write braille. Writing braille by hand requires considerable mental gymnastics, as the page has to be turned over and written on from the rear surface. Politician David Blunkett recalls the difficulty of learning to write braille in the pre-computer era:

> What took so long was that we had to write backwards, from right to left, in mirror image, so that when the paper was turned over the text could be read from left to right as usual. In order not to lose one's place on the large braille sheets, there was a cumbersome wooden frame which was moved down a notch at a time for each fresh line. The stylus had to be pressed hard through the thick paper, and the effort involved caused calluses on the fingers and palms of our small hands. It was all a difficult, frustrating discipline for us cack-handed, lively boys – but what joy it provided in the long run, once we had mastered it.[31]

It is more common today to write braille using a machine such as a Perkins Brailler, a typewriter-like device that pushes dots through the page from the back of a sheet of paper. A brailler comprises six keys, one for each dot in the braille grid. Observing an experienced braillist use one of these machines is a lot like watching a concert pianist, as different combinations of the keys are pressed for each letter, in the same way as playing chords on a piano.

Technology has led to a renaissance in braille use, with the development of electronic braille displays, where metal pins rise and fall to create the braille symbols. Braille readers are no longer dependent on a transcription service and can now access almost any book instantly.

These displays are far more portable and user-friendly than braille books, which are far bulkier than their print versions. The braille version of the first Harry Potter book weighs about 3.5 kilograms, but the paperback version is only about 500 grams.

Print reading

Gordon is frequently told that reading braille is remarkable, usually by someone (like me) who has gazed in amazement as he slides his fingers along a page to read. He counters that it is equally remarkable to be able to read visually, moving the eyes hundreds of times per minute to land at exactly the right point within each word on a page of printed text, then decoding this information into a mental image. It is this process, print reading, that has been at the centre of Gordon's research for more than 40 years. This work is summarised in his 2007 book, *Psychophysics of Reading in Normal and Low Vision*.[32]

Gordon has investigated many problems with reading print experienced by people with vision impairment, which go far beyond the obvious difficulty of not being able to see small characters. Even when words are presented at a large enough size, many times bigger than the visual acuity limit, people with vision impairment tend to read more slowly than their peers with good sight. The reasons for this are complex, such as the fact that fewer letters are seen at one glance (their 'visual span' is smaller),[33] their eye movements are less efficient,[34] their processing speed is slower[35] and they are more reliant on contrast (the print needs to be darker, against a whiter background).[36] People with central vision loss are limited by the reduced efficiency of the peripheral retina, but people with peripheral vision loss find it harder to find their place on a page and to follow a line of text.

As well as identifying the causes of difficulties in reading, Gordon has investigated potential solutions such as presenting words on a computer monitor, one at a time (a technique called 'rapid serial visual presentation', or RSVP),[37] to overcome errors in eye movement control. Scrolled text can be used to help people who are reliant on a small 'window' of healthy vision, a method used by Robin Walker of Royal Holloway, University of London, when he developed his free iPad app 'evReader'. The app helps people with vision impairment to read.[38]

I am often asked whether a particular font is better than any other for people with vision impairment. Some people recommend a font such as Courier, where the letters have a fixed width (so the letter 'i' takes up the same amount of space as the letter 'w'), as this provides more information about the shape of the word. Gordon's work does show some benefit in reading speed when using these fixed-width fonts, but the difference is fairly small as long as the print is large enough.[39] Text size appears to be a far more important factor than the typeface used. Even font types designed for people with low vision, such as the RNIB's Tiresias font, are read at about the same speed when the size is the same.[40]

In an encyclopaedic paper, Gordon worked with the typographer Chuck Bigelow to review the history of print size from the 1400s to the twenty-first century. They show that, with a few exceptions relating to the cost of paper or printing, books have evolved to have a print size that subtends an angle of between 0.2 and 2 degrees at the eye. The paper concludes:

> While economics, ergonomics, technology and functional role of print undoubtedly all influence the choice of print size for particular texts, we conclude that properties of vision constrain the choice to lie within a fluent range of print sizes.[41]

Chuck is a font enthusiast. As one half of the Bigelow and Holmes studio he co-created the Lucida family of fonts, along with Wingdings (which in my experience you only see when your printer has gone wrong). He has the remarkable skill of telling typographic stories as if they were detective thrillers; I don't think many people could make the difference between Times and Times New Roman sound quite so exciting. I've had many pleasurable dinners with Chuck, watching him use a magnifying glass to check the kerning on the font on the menu and criticising the choice of typeface used by a brewery on their craft beer label.

Of course, the size of print that is comfortable to read will depend on the distance at which it is held. In a survey of digital reading, Gordon's student Christina Granquist showed that people with good vision chose a font of height 1mm on a smartphone which is held at 26cm, a letter height of 1.3mm on a tablet computer at 40cm, and a font of 1.4mm for a desktop computer at 52cm.[42] Each of these print sizes subtends an angle of about 2 degrees at the eye (Figure 4.1) – almost exactly the same as the upper limit of the print sizes Gordon Legge and Chuck Bigelow found in their historical paper.

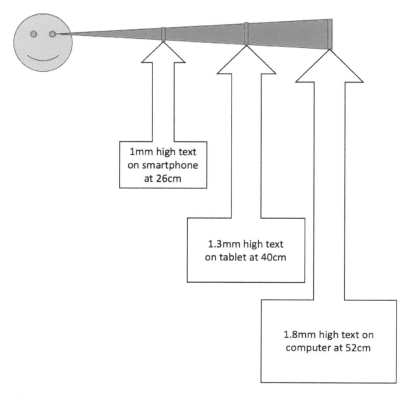

Figure 4.1 Fonts of 1mm at 26cm, 1.3mm at 40cm and 1.8mm at 52cm are the same angular size at the eye. Image drawn by the author.

'Sixth sense'

As well as having better hearing, there is an enduring trope that blind people have a superpower, a sixth sense or ability to see into the future. This belief is at least as old as the Greek myths, where, for example, Tiresias was blinded by the gods as a punishment. Depending on the version of the story you read, this was either because he watched Athena bathing naked, or as the result of an argument between the gods Hera and Zeus over whether men or women enjoy sex more. In this telling of the myth, Tiresias was able to answer the question, as he had been both male and female at different times of his life. He answered 'the woman', to the anger of Goddess Hera, who blinded him. Unable to overcome the punishment of another god, Zeus gave Tiresias the gift of prophecy as compensation for losing his sight. The image of a blind soothsayer persists across time, from Tiresias' appearance in *Oedipus Rex* right up to the twentieth-century Bulgarian clairvoyant Baba Vanga, who allegedly predicted the date of Stalin's death, the Chernobyl disaster and that the forty-fourth president of the USA would be African-American.[43]

This isn't a purely European phenomenon. In Chapter 2, I discussed Zatōichi, the fictional samurai who has appeared in dozens of Japanese books, television series, comics and films since the 1960s. His sixth sense seems to extend to detecting illness. In the first film of the series, he refuses to duel with a rival after correctly identifying that he is dying.

Fairness and justice are popularly associated with blindness, hence Lady Justice being depicted as blindfolded on top of many courthouses, so she can judge without favouring people based on their wealth or appearance.

Echolocation: a true sixth sense?

There is no evidence for blind people being able to prophesy the future, sense disease or communicate with the dead, but there is one sense that some blind people use far more effectively than most people with good vision: echolocation. This is the ability to detect objects by the way in which sounds bounce off them, and is the major way by which bats and dolphins navigate.[44]

In human echolocation, the person makes a noise (such as clicking with their tongue or tapping with a white cane) and interprets the nature of the echo. A quick, hard echo shows a close firm surface, whereas a slowed, muffled reflection suggests a softer, more distant object. Making head movements can also help localise the obstacle, by comparing the volume of the sound in either ear.[45] Echolocation can be trained,[46] although many blind people develop some of these skills spontaneously.

In some circumstances, the world creates sounds so the blind person does not have to make their own noises. In his memoir *Touching the Rock*, John Hull describes standing in his garden during a rainstorm:

> The sound on the path is quite different from the sound of the rain drumming into the lawn on the right, and this is different again from the blanketed, heavy, sodden feel of the large bush on the left … The whole scene is much more differentiated than I have been able to describe, because everywhere are little breaks in the patterns, obstructions, projections, where some slight interruption or difference of texture or of echo gives an additional detail or dimension to the scene.[47]

Later, Hull wishes that it rained always and everywhere: 'If only rain could fall inside a room, it would help me to understand where things are in that room, to give a sense of being in the room, instead of just sitting on a chair.'

The French author and academic Jacques Lusseyran describes this technique as sensing 'vibration', but reports problems with perspective when using this method. On one occasion he recalls thinking a wall was far closer than his guide told him it was, only to realise it was further away but much larger than other walls in the neighbourhood. Lusseyran also writes about how he can sense differences in weather, although he may be detecting atmospheric pressure more than using echolocation.

> What I hear, while leaning out of my window under a grey, overcast sky, is sluggish … The circle in a single plane of space. What I hear when the sun shines has a much more intense vibration.[48]

A non-visual sense of where things are exists in people with perfect sight as well. It's not uncommon to stop abruptly before walking into something despite looking in the opposite direction, and most people could tell if they were in a cathedral or in a cupboard with their eyes closed. Changes in air pressure mean it is quite easy to sense when your hand is hovering just above a table, or when you are standing very close to a wall.

People without sight naturally interact with the world in a different way. Some people with vision impairment have more choices of how to receive information, perhaps choosing braille for poetry, large print for correspondence and audio for textbooks. David Blunkett combines speech and braille: 'I rely far more on cassette tapes than braille, as I can speed the cassette up to get to the point. Reading in braille is a lot slower, but I rely on it where every word is important, as in legislation or important policy papers.'[49] Others use braille to multitask. I've known Gordon to read a braille newspaper discreetly during a concert, although he no longer relies on the braille version of the *New York Times* as its app is now so accessible by using VoiceOver on his iPhone.

Notes

1   Rombaux et al., 2010.
2   Kupers et al., 2011.
3   Renier et al., 2013.
4   Sorokowska, 2016.

5   Sorokowska et al., 2019.
6   Bendas, Hummel and Croy, 2018.
7   Pieniak et al., 2022.
8   Voss et al., 2004.
9   Fieger et al., 2006.
10 Battal et al., 2020.
11 Lewald, 2013.
12 Cappagli, Cocchi and Gori, 2017.
13 Gori et al., 2014.
14 Wan et al., 2010.
15 Hamilton, Pascual-Leone and Schlaug, 2004.
16 Föcker et al., 2012.
17 Liotti, Ryder and Woldorff, 1998.
18 Legge et al., 2008.
19 Oshima et al., 2014.
20 Grant et al., 2016.
21 Ragert et al., 2004.
22 Legge et al., 2019.
23 Frasnelli et al., 2011.
24 Cheung et al., 2009.
25 Nishimura et al., 1999.
26 Heimler, Weisz and Collignon, 2014.
27 Godin, 2021.
28 Mellor, 2006.
29 Holbrook and Zebehazy, 2022.
30 Slade and Edwards, 2015.
31 Blunkett and MacCormick, 2002.
32 Legge, 2007.
33 Legge et al., 1997.
34 Harland, Legge and Luebker, 1998.
35 Cheong et al., 2007.
36 Rubin and Legge, 1989.
37 Rubin and Turano, 1994.
38 Walker et al., 2016.
39 Mansfield, Legge and Bane, 1996.
40 Rubin et al., 2006.
41 Legge and Bigelow, 2011.
42 Granquist et al., 2018.
43 Murray, 2022.
44 Jones, 2005.
45 Stroffregen and Pittenger, 1995.
46 Norman et al., 2021.
47 Hull, 1990.
48 Lusseyran, 1963.
49 Blunkett and MacCormick, 2002.

5
Half the world disappears: brain-related blindness

Sue was watching *Countdown* when she had a stroke. 'The TV's on the blink,' she called to Barry. 'The letters on the side keep coming and going – I can only see four of them.' Barry, a retired telephone engineer, first thought that the signal had been blocked by construction work across the road, where a supermarket was being built. When the TV looked clear to him, he methodically worked through other causes of the problem. He checked Sue's glasses were clean, then made sure she could see his face. 'Something's not right, Barry,' she said. 'I can't see your ear. I've got a bit of a headache too. I think I'd better go for a lie down.'

Barry was worried that Sue might have an eye disease, as several of their friends had age-related macular degeneration, so he phoned the NHS helpline to ask for advice. He thought they were overreacting when they sent an ambulance, and hoped the neighbours weren't worried when it arrived, blue lights flashing, just a few minutes later. Within an hour of watching TV, Sue was having an MRI scan that showed she had experienced a stroke in her left occipital cortex, at the very back of her brain.

Most people know that each side of the body is controlled by the opposite side of the brain. For example, when you touch something with your left hand it is sensed in the right hemisphere, and part of the left hemisphere is responsible for moving your right leg. The visual system works a little differently. Nerves from one eye travel to the visual cortex in both hemispheres, with half of the nerve fibres staying on the same side of the head and the other half crossing over at the optic chiasm in the bottom of the brain. The benefit of this is that we see in 3D and have good hand–eye coordination, but it means that if the visual cortex in one half of the brain is damaged, some of the sight in both eyes is lost.

This is what happened to Sue. The part of her brain that was affected by the stroke enabled her to see the right half of the world with her right eye and also saw the right half of the world from her left eye. After her stroke she had hemianopia, literally 'half sight', so her vision was perfect for everything to her left, but anything to the right of her nose was completely invisible.

Sue was discharged from hospital quickly after her stroke. She was fit and healthy and, as a former teacher, she obediently completed the rehabilitation tasks that were given to her. Her neurologist referred her to the low vision clinic as she thought I might be able to help with some of the problems related to her vision loss. In particular, he thought I might be able to prescribe some prism glasses which would move everything to Sue's left, so she would be more aware of things on her right side.

I looked at Sue and Barry in the waiting room. They were both reading the *Guardian*; Barry had the main part of the paper, and Sue was looking at the supplement. I smiled to myself as I knew from the neurologist's report that Sue wasn't able to read any words at all, but I imagined that after 55 years of marriage the ritual of separating the newspaper this way was fairly hard-wired.

I had arranged the clinic room so that Barry and I were both sitting to Sue's left, as if we were sitting on the other side then she would have had to turn her head uncomfortably to be able to see us. I started by asking about her vision since the stroke. I heard the *Countdown* story and she confirmed that she couldn't read but still liked looking at the newspaper. She told me how she would jump if Barry approached from her right, as he would suddenly appear in front of her, like a jack-in-the-box.

I tested her vision. She could see to the bottom of the visual acuity chart with her glasses but missed the letters to the right of each line. She could read extremely small letters on a reading test, right down to font size four, but couldn't form these letters into words. She could spell the word aloud, but when I asked her what the word was, or what it meant, she shook her head.

Barry had been quiet through the assessment, but I could sense there was something else that was worrying him. I asked what he had noticed about his wife's vision. He replied:

'Well, the neurologist says it's normal, but it's the weirdest thing. She just ignores half of her plate of food; she eats up one side and leaves the rest. It doesn't matter what it is, she just leaves it there. I tell her there's more on her plate and she shouts at me, or looks at me like I've gone crazy.'

The word 'crazy' hung in the air. I wondered if he was concerned that the stroke had done more to Sue's brain than affecting her vision, or whether he thought she might have early signs of dementia. I looked at Sue to see if she would comment but she didn't respond. I wasn't sure if she hadn't heard Barry, or if she was choosing to ignore him.

'A lot of people do the same after a stroke,' I said. 'I saw a man last week who only shaves half of his face every morning, and there are accounts of people who only put lipstick on one side of their lips. It's called "spatial neglect", where not only does the brain not see a part of the world, it actually forgets that it ever existed.' Barry seemed to relax. His shoulders dropped a little, and he smiled. Sue smiled too: 'See, I told you I'm not losing my marbles. This man says it happens all the time!'

Spatial neglect is common following a stroke and doesn't only affect humans. I once had a cat who displayed exactly the same behaviour as Sue. Frank would eat all the biscuits from half of his bowl, licking it clean, and would completely disregard the pile of biscuits on the right. He would call for more food – he had an exceptionally loud miaow – and be grateful when I rotated the bowl through 180 degrees so that he could see and eat the rest of his dinner.

Despite being common, neglect is very hard to conceptualise. We can't see things behind our back, but we still know that the world continues to exist there. Spatial neglect meant that Sue knew intellectually that she couldn't see to her right, but that didn't help. If she didn't know that part of the world existed, how did she know she couldn't see it? When Barry asked her to finish her food, she was as confused as if he had asked her to visit the lost city of Atlantis. For Sue, the rest of the plate just didn't exist.

In one study, researchers asked people with visual neglect to draw a clock face. Most people can draw a pretty accurate clock even with their eyes closed. It might be a bit messy, but it would have all the key details. People with visual neglect might draw half of a perfect clock, as if the other half has just dropped out of their mind (Figure 5.1).

The most extreme form of visual neglect is known as Anton syndrome. In this condition, people get angry when confronted with evidence that they can't see, thinking that people are lying about the part of the world that is invisible to them. Anton syndrome is brilliantly described in Rupert Thomson's novel *The Insult*. This book tells the story of Martin Blom, who is blinded after being shot in the head. Despite strong evidence to the contrary, he starts to believe that he can see, thinking that doctors are lying to him or that he is part of a secret research study. He absconds from hospital and moves to a hotel in the

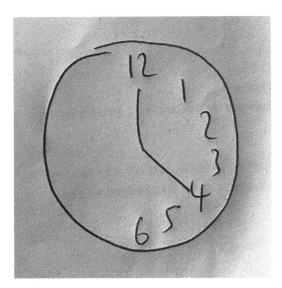

Figure 5.1   An example of how a clock might be drawn by someone with hemispatial neglect. Image drawn by the author.

red-light district of an unidentified European city. Thinking his vision is better at night, he lives a nocturnal existence, eating in late-night cafes and making friends on the fringes of society with a circus knife-thrower, a medically retired trawlerman, an overnight security guard and a dancer from a sleazy bar.

People with Anton syndrome can be very convincing, and Thomson skilfully creates doubt about whether Martin Blom really can see at night or not. It was only on rereading the book that I realised the absence of visual descriptions, as in this portrayal of Leon's, an all-night restaurant:

> You walked in through a rickety glass-and-metal door, passing a curtain that was lined with vinyl to keep out the draughts. Once beyond the curtain you were hit by the smell of sweat and soup and cigarettes … there was a TV in the top corner of the room, its screen angled downwards, like some modern bird of prey. You ate with your eyes fixed on it, one arm curled protectively around your plate.[1]

For me, this passage generates a strong mental image, despite being based largely on non-visual descriptions of touch, sound and smell, which is how the scene is constructed in Blom's head.

Sue's neurologist had wondered whether prism glasses would help her. These glasses can't restore vision, but they can shift the image to one side, moving some things from the unseen area to the healthy part of the visual field. They can stop people bumping into things on their blind side. I have prescribed them to people who use them, for example, in railway stations, in art galleries and at scientific conferences.

Most spectacle lenses focus light without moving the image, but prisms move light in one direction, so the wearer sees the world as if it has shifted to one side. They are most often used to correct adult-onset squints, where the position of one eye suddenly changes. As the eyes are now pointing in different directions, these people usually experience double vision. Putting a prism in front of one eye can move the image so that it is centred with the misaligned eye.

In hemianopia, the prisms are prescribed so that the scene is shifted away from the blind side and towards the healthy side of the visual field. This means that something that falls in to the non-seeing side (for example, a person standing to Sue's right) is seen in the intact part of the visual field, giving time for the wearer to adjust their position and avoid a collision. One of my favourite things to do in the clinic is to stand to the non-seeing side of someone with hemianopia and ask them to take the prism glasses off and on, asking 'Can you see me now? … how about now?' I watch their smile as I appear and disappear from their view.

For many people, the word 'prism' recalls memories of school physics experiments where this type of lens is used to break white light into its constituent colours. This effect is sometimes seen when using prisms for field loss, with people seeing coloured fringes at the edge of the spectacle lens. This isn't always unpleasant, as my patient Sarah reported in a paper we wrote about a new design of prismatic lens:

> One thing I am experiencing though that I didn't expect is rainbows. When I'm outside and the sun is high in the sky (generally just before 1p.m.), I get a vertical rainbow down my vision for a few minutes … it only seems to happen for a few minutes when I'm outside and the sun is really high.[2]

These glasses can work well for people with hemianopia, particularly those without hemispatial neglect. In a randomised controlled trial, about two-thirds of people with hemianopia found them helpful for obstacle avoidance, although some preferred the control prism, perhaps as there were fewer 'rainbows' and other visual phenomena with the sham glasses.[3]

I have found that these glasses particularly help teenagers with hemianopia. Stroke is quite rare in childhood, but hemianopia occurs in children who have had surgery to treat epilepsy. Some children who have very frequent seizures that can't be treated by medication will have a hemispherectomy, a major operation where half of the brain is removed or disconnected. The first human hemispherectomy was performed in 1923 to treat a brain tumour, although physiologists had been experimenting with this operation on animals since the 1880s, with a dog having this operation in 1888. It is reported that the dog kept the same personality with a slight reduction in intelligence.[4]

In about three-quarters of cases, this surgery leads to a child being completely free of seizures, without needing any medication.[5] As the surgery is usually only offered to children having several seizures every day, the improvement in independence and quality of life is remarkable. However, all of these children develop a hemianopia. I am often told that losing part of the visual field is a price worth paying for being able to live without epilepsy.

Jonathan Horton of the University of California, San Francisco, is a world expert in neurology, ophthalmology and physiology. When lecturing, he shows a video of a seven-year-old boy wearing a bright orange San Francisco Giants baseball shirt. The boy introduces himself, hits a baseball very hard, then excitedly runs around a baseball field shouting 'home run!' Following this, Dr Horton shows scans of the boy's brain. The audience gasps as they see that he only has half a functioning brain. Remarkably, the only problem this child experiences are hemianopia, some weakness of one arm and very mild speech impairment.

Vision and the brain

School biology textbooks usually have a detailed anatomical diagram of the eye, showing light being refracted by the cornea, passing through the pupil and lens and forming a perfect inverted image on the retina. The picture usually ends with the optic nerve, perhaps with an arrow saying 'leads to the brain', as if the whole image is sent in its entirety to be recognised. Perhaps understandably, they don't usually go into the phenomenally complex process of breaking down the image into its constituent features and then reconstructing it. The visual areas of the brain do this 1.2 million-piece jigsaw puzzle several times every second, which is one reason why the brain uses so much energy.

After half of the optic nerve fibres cross in the optic chiasm, the first element of processing is in the primary visual cortex, in the occipital lobe at the back of the head. Cells in the primary visual cortex, or V1, respond to features like stripes of different sizes and edges in different orientations. This information is then fed forward, through a series of increasingly specialised visual areas, up to V5. Each region processes different elements of the scene, such as motion in different directions, colours and objects. Beyond V5, visual information interacts with other brain regions linked to functions like memory, reading and movement.

A lot of what is known about the visual system in the brain comes from 'double dissociation' studies. These studies compare people who have had brain injuries in different regions. For example, comparing two people who have had strokes in different parts of their brain, one of whom can read letters but not recognise faces, the other someone who recognises faces but can't read letters, shows the relative importance of these two brain regions for these tasks.

At one time, it was thought that there were specialised cells that existed only for one object, although not all scientists were comfortable with this theory. One paper refers to scientists writing 'with irony about so-called gnostic neurons: the process of recognition begins with spot or line detectors and proceeds till the activation of the "my grandmother" or the "yellow Volkswagen" cell',[6] but now it is thought that brain regions are specialised for groups of images, such as faces. Functional brain imaging shows different levels of activity in these facial areas of the brain (the fusiform face area and the inferior occipital gyrus) in people with prosopagnosia, which is more commonly known as face blindness.[7]

More understanding of how visual processing works in the brain can be obtained by studying visual illusions. Many people will be familiar with the Necker cube illusion, where a simple line drawing of a cube looks to be popping out from the page so either the bottom left face or the top right face appears closer (Figure 5.2). Despite the image in the retina not changing, the direction of the cube seems to 'flip' with extended viewing. This is thought to be caused by decisions made in later visual regions of the brain, which modulate what we see based on the inputs which they receive. The 'flip' occurs when these cells suddenly reinterpret the image that the eye is transmitting.

The Necker cube illusion appears simple but is a source of fascination for some scientists. The scientific database PubMed® shows 241 peer-reviewed published papers on this illusion, examining which parts of the brain are responsible for the illusion,[8,9] determining whether the appearance of the cube can be used as a diagnostic test for dementia[10] and even investigating whether observing the cube can help with problem solving.[11]

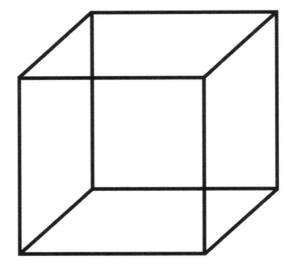

Figure 5.2   The Necker cube. Image drawn by the author.

Visual illusions are sometimes not perceived in the same way by people with diseases like schizophrenia, giving further insights into which brain regions are responsible for these processes, as well as teaching us more about psychiatry.[12,13]

Other brain-related vision impairments

The complexity of the visual system in the brain means that damage or disease to some brain regions can cause unusual visual effects. Palinopsia is a condition where the vision is 'too slow' – once an object has been removed from the visual field it is still seen, a little like a lingering afterimage. Palinopsia can be caused by a wide range of conditions including migraine, drug use and multiple sclerosis.[14]

It can be very difficult for people to explain some unusual visual phenomena and many doctors will assume that the visual system is normal as long as the person has good visual acuity, full visual fields and good colour vision. To address this problem, neuro-ophthalmologists at the National Hospital for Neurology and Neurosurgery in London have developed the 'blue book', a collection of perceptual tests to probe more complex aspects of sight. People are shown this book and asked to perform tasks like differentiating squares from rectangles, identifying objects from photographs taken from unusual angles and recognising famous faces.[15] These tests seem to be sensitive to some of the visual problems associated with dementia, particularly those caused by posterior cortical atrophy (PCA). People with PCA usually have good visual acuity but often report difficulty with visual tasks like counting coins, reading, using a mobile phone or getting dressed.[16] One paper on this condition emphasises to doctors that it is 'important that PCA is considered in late middle-aged patients presenting with progressive visual symptoms and normal visual acuity'. PCA can be a sign of other conditions like Alzheimer disease, Lewy body dementia or Creutzfeldt-Jakob disease.[17]

Although awareness of PCA among doctors and optometrists is increasing (the College of Optometrists in the UK, in particular, provides continuing education sessions on this disease), it is still common to meet professionals unaware of the condition. Here someone with PCA eloquently expresses their frustration when medical staff repeatedly failed to identify their condition:

> I was constantly being bumped from pillar to post either at the hospital ophthalmic department or another trying to work out why I couldn't read properly and everything was falling off ... things would slide off the page, I would say like icing off a cake.[17]

Visual hallucinations in blindness

One consequence of the way the brain's visual system is organised is that it doesn't always respond well to an absence of information, which happens when part of the eye stops working. In some cases, this absence of input can cause cells in higher visual regions of the brain to respond inappropriately, creating a false image to be seen – a hallucination. Visual hallucinations related to blindness are often referred to as Charles Bonnet hallucinations, named after the eighteenth-century Swiss scientist who first identified this phenomenon in his 89-year-old grandfather, Charles Lullin.[18] Lullin had advanced cataracts in both eyes, disrupting his visual system. He experienced elaborate visual hallucinations, including detailed images of 'men, women, birds, carriages and buildings'.[19] Charles Bonnet correctly identified that these visions were not associated with dementia or psychiatric disease. For many years, Charles Bonnet syndrome was said to occur in 'the elderly with intact cognition',[19] although it is now known to affect children and young people with eye disease as well.[20]

An important way to differentiate Charles Bonnet syndrome (CBS) from other causes of hallucination, like psychosis, dementia or Parkinson's disease, is that the person experiencing them knows they are imaginary. They will not attempt to start a conversation with a hallucinated face or open a window to let the hallucinatory bird escape.

In the low vision clinic, I tend to ask whether people have experienced hallucinations at the end of the examination, when I hope to have achieved a rapport. I usually mention CBS factually: 'Sometimes people with eye diseases like yours see things that aren't there, as their brain tries to fill in the gaps in their vision but sometimes gets it wrong,' then stay quiet for a few seconds. About one time in 10, the silence will be broken with something along the lines of 'I'm so glad you said that – I thought I was losing my mind!' They follow with a description of balloons, flowers, faces or dogs that they have hallucinated.

The fear of dementia and mental illness is so strong that it is hard to work out the real prevalence of this syndrome. Even on very careful and tactful questioning it is natural that some people will not admit to seeing things that aren't there. At least one-third of people with sight loss do report hallucinations,[21] although the true proportion is probably much higher. Despite being so common, CBS is still not widely known about, even by doctors. In 2018, a survey of Canadian family physicians found that more than half knew nothing about it.[22] In the UK, the charity Esme's Umbrella works with doctors and people with sight loss to increase awareness of the condition, reducing the stigma associated with seeing things that aren't there.[23]

Several strategies can help to overcome CBS, including blinking, making eye movements, walking around, looking at lights or trying to touch the image.[24] In more serious cases, counselling, cognitive behavioural therapy or drug treatment can be used, with antipsychotic,[25] anti-epileptic[26] or serotonin reuptake inhibitor drugs sometimes helping.[27] Even without treatment, the hallucinations tend to reduce over time. In about one third of people, they disappear completely within one year and the frequency of seeing them decreases in another 20 per cent.[21] Sometimes reassurance is enough to reduce the impact of CBS on people's quality of life.

Blindsight

Another unusual visual phenomenon experienced by some people with sight loss is blindsight. This refers to the ability of some people to respond correctly to a question about a visual scene (for example, 'Is this striped pattern horizontal or vertical?', or 'Is this letter an X or an O?') without being able to see it.[28] In an early description of blindsight, from 1974, Weiskrantz and colleagues described a man with complete hemianopia who could perform these tasks in his blind field with about 90 per cent accuracy, despite not being aware of 'seeing' the targets at all.[29] This is a key feature of blindsight: the person does not perceive the target, but when forced to guess at an answer (X or O, for example) they are nearly always right.

Blindsight is rare. Despite meeting people with hemianopia about once a month in the clinic, I have not yet seen anyone who I have been convinced has this phenomenon. It is thought to be caused by alternative neural pathways from the eye which bypass the visual areas of the brain, similar to those that are used in sleep regulation, although the question of 'why blindsight is blind' (and not perceived) is still debated.[30]

Non-organic vision loss

So far I have described how brain disease causes vision impairment, how the brain can create images when nothing is there and how the brain can sometimes see without being aware of seeing. To end this chapter, I will discuss people who don't see things despite the eyes and brain being completely healthy – those with non-organic vision loss.

A simple case of non-organic vision loss would be someone who can see well but would like to wear glasses. Most optometrists will have met primary-school age children whose best friends have just been prescribed glasses and who would like some themselves. By claiming not to see, they assume they will also get some spectacles. This is usually quite easy for an experienced optometrist to determine; for example, sometimes they say they can see nothing at all until a zero-power plain glass lens is placed in front of the eye, at which point they will read the bottom line of the chart. Reassurance that the eyes are completely healthy and perhaps the opportunity to get sunglasses is usually enough to address this situation.

People sometimes claim to have poor sight to account for difficulties in other areas of their life. I have seen this many times in children who are not living up to their parents' expectations educationally, particularly teenagers in high-pressure schools who are cramming for exams, for whom claiming not to see well can be a convenient excuse for falling behind. Sometimes this is quite easy to determine due to inconsistency in the eye examination. For example, they consistently might read only the top line of a sight chart, regardless of the distance at which the chart is held, which doesn't make sense (they should be able to see letters of half the size from half the distance). Alternatively, they might say that they can't see letters smaller than font size 48 on a reading test, but be able to read a message on their smartwatch displayed in font size 10. A particularly devious way to uncover this type of inconsistency is to ask the teenager to pick something up, like a small sweet or a dropped pen, and see how accurately they can do this.

Managing someone with this type of vision loss requires empathy and very careful explanation. I am pleased that the horrible term 'malingering' has fallen out of favour, although some of my colleagues still use this outdated word. Non-organic, functional or medically unexplained vision loss are far more appropriate descriptions.

Non-organic vision loss can also reflect psychological trauma. An investigation of 15 adolescents with this condition found that 11 of them had experienced bereavement in the previous year and that nearly half had been bullied.[31] In extreme cases, non-organic vision loss can be a linked to sexual assault, abuse or neglect. Care for people with non-organic vision loss can require the input of many non-ophthalmic professionals such as paediatricians, counsellors, therapists and psychiatrists. One psychologist working with children with vision impairment told me that she has seen a huge rise in the number of young people with anxiety-related non-organic sight loss since the start of the coronavirus pandemic. This group of people now makes up nearly half of her caseload.

Some eye conditions can be extremely hard to detect, particularly in their early stages, so non-organic vision loss is only diagnosed when there is evidence that the person can definitely see at a normal level. In some cases, this is confirmed using electrophysiological testing where the tiny electrical signals in the brain that respond to visual targets are measured carefully.

It is important to emphasise that non-organic vision loss can be as 'real' as vision loss from glaucoma, a stroke or any other disease, and that it is as genuine as having a rash or a fever. In the low vision clinic, I approach people with this type of blindness in the same way as someone with any other cause of vision impairment. I find that the same strategies (like magnification, contrast enhancement, tinted glasses or eye movement training) can help. Pleasingly, non-organic vision loss tends to improve with time.

Non-organic disorders are also seen in other parts of medicine. Consultant neurologist Suzanne O'Sullivan's excellent book *It's All in Your*

Head: True Stories of Imaginary Illness describes people who experience psychogenic grand mal seizures with no brain disease. As well as being a superb writer, Dr O'Sullivan is clearly an empathetic and caring clinician who would never describe someone with this life-impacting condition as 'a malingerer'.[32]

* * *

Sue's visual neglect improved over the next few months, although she is still completely blind to her right. Prism glasses didn't work for her, but she has made other changes. Barry took my advice to rearrange the living room so that the television is to her left, when they go out he always walks on her right to fend off obstacles, and he rotates Sue's dinner plate without speaking. She has been using a computer rehabilitation program called Read-Right, which means she can read short words now, although it is still frustratingly slow for her, so she and Barry have started listening to audiobooks. She has learnt to play *Countdown* in her head rather than relying on what she sees on the screen and she no longer shouts at Barry when he points out something that she's forgotten about. Her life now is a little different to before her stroke, but with these adaptations Sue is still active and fulfilled.

Notes

1   Thomson, 1996.
2   Crossland, Reuben and Bedford, 2022.
3   Bowers, Keeney and Peli, 2014.
4   Kenneally, 2006.
5   Griessenauer et al., 2015.
6   Velichkovsky and Zinchenko, 1982.
7   Hadjikhani and de Gelder, 2002.
8   Kornmeier and Bach, 2005.
9   Loued-Khenissi and Preuschoff, 2020.
10   Fernandez-Viadero, Crespo and Verduga, 2000.
11   Laukkonen and Tangen, 2017.
12   Dakin, Carlin and Hemsley, 2005.
13   Notredame et al., 2014.
14   Schimansky, Bennetto and Harrison, 2022.
15   Kim et al., 2021.
16   Keuss, Bowen and Schott, 2019.
17   Bowen et al., 2019.
18   Ffytche, 2007.
19   Ffycthe, 2005.
20   Jones and Moosajee, 2021.
21   Jackson, Bassett and Nirmalan, 2005.
22   Gordon and Felfeli, 2018.
23   Esme's Umbrella, accessed 11 October 2022.
24   Best et al., 2019.

25   Coletti Moja et al., 2005.

26   Paulig and Mentrip, 2001.

27   Lang et al., 2007.

28   Danckert, Striemer and Rossetti, 2021.

29   Weiskrantz et al., 1974.

30   Stoerig and Cowey, 2007.

31   Wynick, Hobson and Jones, 1997.

32   O'Sullivan, 2016.

6
The heinous sin of self-pollution: guilt, denial and the psychology of blindness

Jay's approach to losing his sight – perhaps his approach to life in general – is to joke about it and tell anecdotes. A large man in his mid-twenties, he has a plume of unruly red hair and wears immaculately tailored suits. He is a great storyteller with a contagious laugh, and I always smile when I see his name on the clinic list. Jay attends the hospital because he has retinitis pigmentosa – a serious retinal disease that is gradually but irrevocably leading him to total blindness.

In the low vision clinic a couple of years ago, I was laughing at one of Jay's stories – this one about mistakenly getting into a waiter's car rather than his partner's – when his face fell. He looked towards his shoes and said, in a quiet voice, 'Do you think it's because I masturbated a lot as a teenager?' The heat from his blushing face radiated across the consultation room.

I moved my chair slightly closer to his, mirrored his concerned expression and tried to hide my surprise at the sudden turn in the conversation.

'What makes you say that?' I asked. 'You know we think this is inherited.' Modern genetic testing meant that Jay knew exactly which gene – RPGR – caused his vision loss. He had a grandfather with the same condition, now completely blind. Jay stuttered a little. 'I know. It's just … I can't help thinking … when I was 14, my eyes started going bad and …' His voice trailed off.

Serious eye disease often develops in people's teens and our brains are hard-wired to create associations. If a disease develops at the same time as a new habit, then it is natural to assume the two events are linked. This is especially true if we are told the habit is harmful. Jay was brought up in a Catholic family, and probably knew the catechism that says masturbation is an 'intrinsically and gravely disordered action'.[1]

'You're not the first person to ask me this,' I told Jay, 'but do you know where that belief comes from?' This gave me the excuse to turn the tables and tell Jay one of my own favourite stories. In the early eighteenth century, a book was published with the fabulous title *Onania: or, the Heinous Sin of Self-Pollution, and All its Frightful Consequences (in Both Sexes) Consider'd; With Spiritual and Physical Advice to Those who Have already Injur'd themselves by this Abominable Practice*.[2] Believed to have been written by quack physician John Marten,[3] the book was so popular that, by 1730, it was in its fifteenth printing, although it was being sold by a different publisher, with the cover stating that 'Mr Crouch, bookseller, who us'd also to sell it, being dead'.

'Dimness of sight' is the most enduring myth from *Onania*, but Marten described dozens of other associated conditions, including growth retardation, epilepsy, gonorrhoea, depression and memory loss. More pornographer than physician, Marten's book includes dozens of raunchy testimonials written by people describing their experiences of masturbation-induced illness. Titillating passages describe the behaviour of 'lascivious widows' and misbehaving schoolgirls. Readers are told that redemption comes from abstinence, prayer and frequent doses of 'strengthening tincture', conveniently sold by John Marten.

Marten was not the only doctor in town profiting from attitudes to masturbation. William Farrer also sold remedies for those afflicted by the consequences of this habit. In his 1767 book *A Short Treatise on Onanism*, he describes some ophthalmological features of a frequent masturbator:

> when he was about to read any thing, he seemed to be drunk, and flushed with wine; the pupils of his eyes were extremely dilated, and his eyes themselves racked with darting pains, accompanied with some degree of tension; … both corners of his eyes … were also clogged and stuffed with a whitish kind of matter.[4]

Although Marten and his peers were charlatans, more respected doctors shared the belief that masturbation could lead to poor sight. In an early example of a literature review, celebrated physician Samuel-Auguste Tissot described several cases of poor sight associated with what he called 'secret and excessive venery', ranging from gutta serena (blindness of unknown cause, also known as amaurosis) to 'a langour in the eyes' and the vision being 'bleared'.[5]

There were other reasons why people associated poor vision with poor behaviour. Before antibiotics, sailors frequently went blind due to syphilis. Pubic lice infestation caused people's eyelashes to fall out. It is no surprise that blindness has long been equated with immorality.

Jay sticks in my memory, but I have met people who associated all sorts of innocent activities with poor vision. Blindness caused by overuse of the eyes is a particularly long-standing belief. 350 years ago, the poet John Milton wrote: 'From the twelfth year of my age I scarcely ever went from my lessons to bed before midnight; which indeed was the first cause of injury to my eyes.'[6] Nearly every week I will hear someone say: 'If only I hadn't read so much as a child,' or 'I wish I hadn't watched TV with the lights off.'

The fear of blindness is so strong that it can be used as a parenting tool. I am frequently asked to tell children to spend less time on their iPad because it's 'bad for their eyes' (it's not, or at least it's no worse than reading a book). Older colleagues tell me they were asked the same thing about videos, and before that colour television was seen as somehow more harmful than black and white. I am waiting for the first time I meet someone who blames their blindness on too much time spent in virtual reality. There are no harmful rays emitted from electronic displays and even the brightest computer screen is far less bright than the sky on an overcast day. Some people can experience eye strain from focusing at one distance for a prolonged period of time and there is a link between excessive close work and developing myopia, but screens, televisions and videos are not inherently dangerous.

Jay knew that his eye disease was genetic, so why blame himself for his blindness? Health beliefs are complex – people often take Western and Chinese medicines simultaneously, or continue with prescribed medication when making a pilgrimage to Lourdes. It is completely plausible to believe in genetics and the sins of self-pollution. Guilt is a common response to losing sight, and it is this emotion which John Marten and his peers exploited to financial gain.

Like many lies, there is a tiny grain of truth in the association between masturbation and sight loss. The Valsalva manoeuvre is a sudden rise in pressure in the chest, caused by attempting to exhale while the airways are closed. Sometimes people do this deliberately, such as when they hold their nose and blow out to try and cure a blocked ear after getting off an aeroplane. This pressure rise can also be caused by heavy lifting, vomiting, straining to defecate or, in rare cases, masturbation or sex.[7],[8] Very occasionally, this leads to preretinal bleeding, which can obstruct the vision. When describing this phenomenon, modern authors appear keen to avoid the titillation that Marten's book was prone to. In one case series of six people with vision loss associated with sexual activity, the raciest phrases are 'a variant of heterosexual intercourse', 'arousal with a handheld massage machine' and 'particularly vigorous autoerotic activity'. The paper opens with the puritanical phrase 'Sexual activity is associated with many perils.'[9]

Valsalva-associated vision loss generally affects only one eye and is resolved on its own, as the blood is reabsorbed. This is very different to Jay's experience of blindness, but may have been one of the origins of the myth that 'it makes you go blind'.

Denial

As well as guilt, denial can be part of the psychological process of losing sight. Recently, I met Mina, a 28-year-old woman whose vision was progressively getting worse due to a different inherited disease. She was finding it difficult to see small details. Her work in the head office of a bank was getting more difficult and she had recently ruined her dinner because she read '30 minutes' as '50 minutes' in a recipe book. She assumed new glasses would help and was quite angry when I explained that I couldn't improve on the spectacles she had been using for a few years. I suggested that she might want to use other devices that could help her see more easily and showed her a few low vision aids to magnify print. She discounted the first magnifying glass I showed her as too small, yet the larger one I showed her was 'too heavy'. Each time I found a different device that might help there was a new problem – one of them was too strong, one cast a shadow on the page, another one made her feel dizzy. When I suggested that her occupational health department in the bank might be able to recommend a larger monitor, she said: 'Yes, but it will be too bright for me if it's bigger. There must be something you can do with these – can't you try again?', waving her hand at the 250 lenses in the trial case I'd used to test her eyes.

I recognised this pattern. One of my mentors, Liz Gould, recommended a few books to me when I first started working in the low vision clinic. I remember being surprised that the first book she recommended, *Games People Play* by Eric Berne, made no mention of blindness, or eyesight at all.[10] Instead it described human interactions and communication, which is the most fundamental part of my work. Some now dismiss Berne's work as 1960s pop psychology, and some of the language has dated, but it was this book that I drew on in

Mina's consultation, as I realised she was playing Berne's 'Why Don't You – Yes But' game. Each suggestion I made was met with rejection. Dr Berne suggests responding to the 'Yes But' game by moving to another game, which he calls 'Rapo', by closing the conversation and moving on. Although I don't think about it in game terms, my experience is that there's no benefit in continuing to try and problem-solve in this situation. 'I'm glad you've seen these magnifiers,' I told Mina. 'They might not be right for you yet, but keep them in mind, and just let me know if you want to look at them again. They might become useful one day.'

I only had to wait about three weeks before an email pinged on my screen, with Mina's name and hospital number as the subject. One of the departmental clerks had written: 'Hi Michael. This lady called, she would like to look at the magnifiers you showed her again, can you advise her what to do?' After a relatively straightforward assessment, Mina left with a small folding magnifier with an LED light for her pocket, a larger one with a light for her kitchen and a letter to her employer asking them to reassess her workspace.

Sight loss and the grieving process

Denial is often cited as being the first stage of the grieving process. In Elisabeth Kübler-Ross's well-known 'five stages of grief' model, denial is followed by anger, bargaining, depression and acceptance. Although the model is often used to describe people's response to bereavement, Kübler-Ross developed it after observing people with life-limiting disease.[11] This has led psychologists to apply this model to losing vision, or any other sense. In an entertaining and detailed description of the grieving process of losing his vision, Professor of English Chris Mounsey gives examples of his behaviour at each stage of this process: from denial ('I was in denial about the problems with my sight for so long that I even learned to drive a car, and my lousy driving caused most of the major arguments in my life'); anger ('now I apologise to everyone I've upset with my intransigent stare through the hard surfaces of my sunglasses'); bargaining ('here's the bargain: if I can see half as well, I'll work twice as hard'); depression ('when you work to stave off the fear of grieving, the cycle of depression spirals ever downward'); and acceptance ('accept my new self and put behind me my grieving for the old self').[12]

The grieving process doesn't always follow this linear pattern and Kübler-Ross's stages of grief are far from universal, but it is common for me to meet people in the clinic who are clearly at one of these stages. My work is easiest during consultations with people who accept their vision loss and who are willing to accept new approaches to tackling visual tasks, but in most clinics I will meet someone with vision impairment who has some signs of depression.

Mental health in vision impairment

Depression is very common. About 10 per cent of people have some form of depression at any given time,[13–15] and about one in three people has an episode of depression at some point in their lifetime.[16] Depression appears to be even more common in people with sight loss. One recent study of adults with low vision found that 43 per cent of people attending low vision clinics had significant symptoms of depression, of whom only a quarter were receiving treatment.[17]

A common way for screening for depression in a medical appointment is to use the Patient Health Questionnaire-2, which asks two questions:[18]

- Over the last two weeks, how often have you been bothered by having little interest or pleasure in doing things?
- Over the last two weeks, how often have you been bothered by feeling down, depressed or hopeless?

Responses of 'more than half the days' to one question, and at least 'several days' to the other, raise the possibility of depression and should lead to more detailed questioning. However, there is a chance that these questions might overdiagnose depression in people with vision impairment. Some people will respond 'every day' to the first question, not because they have depression but because they can't take pleasure from an activity that they can no longer see to do. If someone has spent decades doing a cryptic crossword over breakfast, but their sight has stopped them from doing it, they may be bothered by having little pleasure in doing this activity, without necessarily being depressed.

Even with this caveat, it is clear that depression is a problem for many people with sight loss, and it does not only affect the person with vision impairment. In a study of 418 married couples, Strawbridge and colleagues showed people with a vision-impaired spouse were also at increased risk of depression.[19] Women married to visually impaired men were more likely to have depression than men who are married to women with vision impairment, perhaps due to the increased burden of care placed on women. A change in the health of one partner can challenge the sense of 'we-ness' in a romantic relationship and can limit activities that couples previously enjoyed together.[20] In a study of couples where one partner has lost their vision, 'Roy' described the impact of vision loss on eating dinner together:

> It's a moment of sharing, absolutely. We first have the aperitif; we drink a good bottle of wine. And then, we prepare the meal. And then, well, we hang out at the table … I was afraid we would talk about my eyes at our meals, so I tended to avoid them, I spent less time at the table.[20]

Anxiety and mental ill-health

Depression and anxiety are closely linked, with about 85 per cent of people with depression having significant anxiety and 90 per cent of people with anxiety showing some signs of depression,[21] so it is unsurprising that there is a higher rate of anxiety in people with vision impairment.[22]

Fear of losing vision can be related to being anxious. In a longitudinal study, Charles Frank and colleagues examined the rate of depression, anxiety and vision impairment in 7,500 older adults living in the USA.[22] They found a bidirectional relationship – people with vision loss were more likely to develop depression and anxiety, but people with anxiety were also more likely to become visually impaired over the course of the study. Dr Frank suggests several reasons for anxiety preceding vision impairment. He suggests that people who are anxious before losing their vision might be anxious because they have been diagnosed with a serious eye condition, because they have a strong family history of a blinding eye disease, or because they have another health condition, such as diabetes or multiple sclerosis, which then causes vision loss. He also points out that people with anxiety might lose vision due to bad habits (such as a poor diet) or because they are less likely to present to a doctor or optometrist to seek eye care.[22]

Some people with vision impairment also develop post-traumatic stress disorder (PTSD).[23] Researchers from the Netherlands interviewed people with sight loss who had PTSD and found that this condition can be linked to traumatic events associated with having poor vision, such as traffic accidents, falls and even abuse.[24]

Untreated depression is a huge public health issue. The risk of suicidal ideation (giving 'serious thought' to taking your own life), of having plans for committing suicide and of attempting suicide are increased for people with vision loss.[25] However, it is thought that vision impairment alone is not sufficient to cause suicide, and that a combination of hopelessness and vision loss is the mechanism behind these attempts. There are other risk factors for suicide that are indirectly associated with vision loss, such as other health conditions, socio-economic disparities, loneliness and unmet mental health needs.[25,26]

Suicidal ideation can be part of Kübler-Ross's grieving process on losing vision and the vast majority of those who think about suicide don't take their own life. Reassuringly, there is no evidence that the death rate from suicide is higher among people with vision loss compared to the wider population.[27] Early identification of people at risk of suicide, along with prompt access to treatment and counselling support, is key to reducing this small risk even further[28] and counselling services for adults and children with vision impairment have multiplied in recent years. In the UK, the Macular Society, Royal National Institute of Blind People and hospital eye departments offer this support, as do many other services.

Treatment of mental health conditions in people with vision impairment

Although some research has found only a quarter of people with vision impairment and depression were receiving formal treatment,[17] it is likely that many of them were taking other actions to improve their mental health. Few people would think of going for a walk or having a gossip with a neighbour as 'treatment', yet exercise and human contact are effective methods of preventing and treating depression[15,29–32] and anxiety.[33–35] Outdoor exercise seems to be particularly beneficial.[36] The relationship between physical activity and better mental health seems even more marked in people with vision impairment.[37] The 'Inclusive Fitness Initiative' in the UK is working to increase access to gyms and fitness centres for people with all types of disability, although progress has been slow in recruiting venues for this scheme.[38]

Current management of depression is based on a matched-care approach, where the type of treatment is based on the severity of disease, past experiences of treatment and patient preference. The first stage is active monitoring and support, then talking therapies. If the condition is more severe, then medication, crisis services, electroconvulsive therapy and inpatient treatment might be used.[39] A similar stepped-care model, including cognitive behavioural therapy and problem-solving treatment, is effective at preventing depression and anxiety from developing in the first place in people with visual impairment,[40] which suggests that counselling should be offered to everyone with vision loss. I find that people are far more open to talking about their mental health than when I first started working in the low vision clinic in the 1990s. Teenagers are particularly receptive to the idea of counselling, probably as schools have done so much to reduce the stigma around mental illness.

Depression in vision impairment, and its treatment, is one of the main themes of low vision conferences and research is examining the impact of interventions as diverse as having pets, mentoring and art therapy. I am currently working on a Macular Society-funded project, examining what support can be offered to teenagers with inherited macular disease, called STOMP (Supporting Teenagers to Overcome Macular Problems). Our approach will be to design a support package based on what people with lived experience of inherited macular disease tell us they find helpful, rather than the current model of 'doctor knows best', where people are referred to see a counsellor, a low vision clinic or a peer support network only if the clinician thinks it would help.

Breaking bad news

Counsellors talk about the 'point of impact' when coming to terms with vision loss. For some people, this is when they receive the diagnosis of a sight-threatening condition, for others it's when they sign the forms to be registered as severely sight impaired, but for many people it's when they're told that they can no longer drive.

I recently heard the story of a motorcycle policeman who was involved in a road collision. As he didn't see the car that hit him (until it was too late), he was sent to the police force's occupational health doctor who arranged an urgent appointment at a hospital eye department. After the eye examination, the ophthalmologist told him that he had advanced glaucoma and that his visual field was severely reduced. His 'point of impact' was at that first appointment, when the doctor asked him: 'How did you get here?' After hearing 'I drove. My car's in the car park,' the doctor simply said: 'Well, you're not driving home.' The policeman obediently got the bus home. The following day he went to the police station, saw his chief inspector and handed in his badge, saying 'There's no way I can work anymore.'

The story, eventually, has a happier ending. The policeman in question now works for a charity supporting young people who have had similar experiences. I hope that the policeman's ophthalmologist realised how callous his statement was and reflected on how he could break bad news more sensitively in the future. The consultation was in the 1980s, but I am not convinced that things are any better now. Doctors still receive remarkably little teaching in communication skills.

In a recent paper entitled 'It was Like Being Hit by a Brick …', Anne Ferrey and colleagues from Oxford interviewed 18 people and asked about their experiences of being told they had a serious eye disease.[41] The title of the paper comes from a quotation from one patient, who they called Margaret:

> He said to me 'Right … there's no point in beating about the bush … You're blind' … It was like being hit with a brick.

A theme which they identified was the convoluted process of reaching a diagnosis, with the final result coming out of the blue. For example, 'Colin' said: 'I had a few eye tests. Nobody would ever tell me what the eye tests were related to. But, eventually, after one set of eye tests in early 1999, I got the letter, a four-line letter, saying that I had retinitis pigmentosa, I was below the required limit for driving. I had to hand my licence in. And that was it.'

It was clear from Dr Ferrey's research that people preferred having bad news broken to them in person rather than by letter, but it was also important that the clinicians didn't pity their patients too much. One participant stated:

> He looked at me, sort of shook his head and he said 'You poor, poor boy' and … that has actually stayed with me my whole life … (it) really made me feel like it was something incredibly bad … it sort of tainted my view … of the condition.

At the same time, it is important that people aren't dismissed and treated with too little emotion, as 'Betty' says:

> I was told in no uncertain terms by the doctors – quite callously, I thought … 'the sight's gone in that eye, cells have been damaged beyond repair', 'that's gone, forget that'. That was actually said to me.

It is a difficult balance for clinicians between being too matter-of-fact and too pitying. I have been taught that it is important to be empathetic rather than sympathetic, to say 'this must be extremely difficult' rather than 'oh, you poor thing,' but I do wonder if I sometimes fall on the side of being too businesslike. I have worked with consultants with phenomenal communication skills. As well as being a world expert in retinal disease since the 1970s, Professor Alan Bird was an exemplary communicator. At his retirement party in the early 2000s, one of his patients said: 'He was so kind, I almost didn't mind him telling me I was going blind.'

Is depression normal in people with vision impairment?

A question that psychologists often ask people is: 'How much does this bother you?' I often meet people who have a low mood but acknowledge that this is a natural response to losing their eyesight. It is understandable and common to feel bad about any health condition, particularly one that limits the activities that can be performed. In many ways, I am more concerned by people with poor vision who seem completely unfazed by their sight loss, as this might mean they are still in a stage of denial.

I find that listening to people's concerns and explaining that low mood and anxiety is a natural response to losing any sense is very much valued by people in the clinic, particularly those who have recently experienced a 'point of impact'. Very often, people who I see in the clinic who have low mood are almost transformed when I see them again a few months later – they are more stoic, more willing to accept help and often happier, seeing vision impairment as another part of life's rich tapestry.

Does blindness protect against some psychiatric disorders?

Not every mental health condition is more common in people with sight loss. Schizophrenia is very rare in those who are born with severe vision impairment. In fact, there has never been a reported case of schizophrenia in someone who has been severely vision impaired from birth.[42-44] This is thought to be due to changes in the way the brain processes information in the absence of sight, which are protective against psychosis.

This effect was first noticed in the 1950s and was presented in the gendered language typical of the time:

The means required for coping with schizophrenic patients who are also blind would tend to make them memorable. Yet men who had treated more than ten thousand patients had difficulty recalling one who was blind.[45]

Some researchers have suggested that as schizophrenia and congenital cortical blindness are both quite rare (about 0.5 per cent of people have schizophrenia and even fewer are blind from birth), it might be that the coincidence of these two conditions is so rare that it hasn't been noticed by psychiatrists.[46] However, since 1950, millions of patients have been assessed by hundreds of thousands of psychiatrists. Given that many doctors are very keen to publish case reports on their patients (and that a report of schizophrenia in a blind person would be newsworthy), it seems likely that this effect is real.

'Real' guilt in blindness

Jay probably felt guilty as part of the psychological process related to losing his vision, but some blind people are found guilty by a law court for reasons unconnected to their vision loss.

James wasn't a reliable attender of hospital appointments. He'd come for consultations regularly for a few months, then his record would show a swathe of missed visits. It took me a while to realise that the times he didn't attend were because he was in prison.

James had always had poor vision. He was born prematurely and needed laser treatment to save his sight when he was just a few days old. Like many children born early, he developed an extreme form of shortsightedness and needed thick glasses from the age of two. He never liked wearing glasses and, despite the fact that he could see virtually nothing without spectacles, his records from the children's clinic showed that he usually came to appointments without his glasses, having broken or 'lost' them.

The first series of missed appointments was when James was about 14 years old and discovered he preferred flirting, smoking cannabis and stealing cars to sitting in classrooms or reading books. It would be charitable to attribute James's school record to his sight loss, but when I asked him whether he thought not being able to see was related to skipping school, he laughed at me:

Nah, mate, I'm just a bad 'un. People like you, you're always going to go to school, blind or not. I could have had the sight of an eagle but ask me if I'd rather go to school or go out nicking things from Sainsbury's and I'd be down the shops in a flash. It's just how it is!

James certainly looked the part of a bad 'un: his forearms were covered in inexpert tattoos, he had a few missing teeth and he looked at least 10 years older than his age. He carried a faint air of tobacco and whisky, and picked at his teeth with his little fingernail when thinking.

I enjoy James's appointments. Nothing makes him hurry. He ambles rather than walks, and he is clearly interested in people. He always asks me as many questions as I ask him – about my family, other people I've seen with eye conditions like his and what I'm working on at the moment.

I think James sees himself as a loveable rogue, in the vein of the Artful Dodger. I have no idea what he's been in prison for (it would be irrelevant and inappropriate to ask), but I do know his criminal career is frequently thwarted by his eyesight. He once told me the story of one of his many arrests:

> Everyone scarpered, and it was just muggins here who got nicked. I tried to leg it but didn't realise I was running straight towards the police van. That copper must have thought it was Christmas when I ran straight into his arms. Must have been the easiest arrest he'll ever make!

Born 60 years before James, Jacques Lusseyran also had eye problems related to being very shortsighted. A shortsighted eye is 'too long or too strong'; either the eye is larger than average, or the cornea is more steeply curved than normal. In either case, people can't see clearly more than a few centimetres away, hence 'short sighted'. Although most people with myopia go through life with few eye problems beyond needing glasses or contact lenses, a bigger eye is more prone to sight-threatening conditions like maculopathy, glaucoma and retinal detachment. Retinal detachment can be spontaneous, but for both James and Jacques it was caused by trauma: through a pub fight in James's case and a childhood accident in Jacques's. Jaques Lusseyran had the misfortune of suffering from sympathetic ophthalmia. Injury in one eye caused a serious, sight-threatening inflammation in the other, leading to total blindness in both eyes.

Lusseyran's childhood couldn't be more different to James's. He was a scholarly child and had a privileged upbringing in Paris. At lycée he particularly enjoyed philosophy and excelled at languages. In his autobiography *And There Was Light*, Lusseyran describes running across the Champ de Mars, and walking through the Jardin du Luxembourg on his way to school.[47]

Lusseyran was seven years old when he lost his sight and he is almost unbelievably dismissive of the effect this had on him. For example, in this passage he makes blindness sound slightly less significant than a bad cold:

> Blinded on 3 May, by the end of the month I was walking again. In June I began learning to read in Braille. In July I was on a beach on the Atlantic, hanging by the trapeze, by the rings and sliding down the slides.

In defiance of those who think the Kübler-Ross model is the universal response to sight loss, Lusseyran describes the accident that caused his blindness with no malice or anger.

> At ten o'clock I jumped up with my classmates, who were running for the door to the playground outside. In the scuffle, an older boy who was in a hurry came up from the back of the room and ran into me accidentally from behind. I hadn't seen him coming and, taken off guard, lost my balance and fell. As I fell, I struck one of the sharp corners of the teacher's desk.

Lusseyran clarifies that the collision was accidental and empathises with the older boy being in a hurry. Today I might think that these phrases were the result of counselling, and that a therapist had worked through this traumatic event, but I think this reflects Jacques Lusseyran's positive demeanour. He continues:

> Every day since then I have thanked heaven for making me blind when I was still a child not quite eight years old … I am deeply moved when I think of all the people whom blindness strikes when they are fully grown, whether it is caused by accident or injury in war. Often they have a hard lot, certainly one harder than mine.

In common with many blind people, Lusseyran developed a love of radio. Coupled with his language skills, this made him very aware of the threat of France being invaded. After the fall of Paris, he was quick to join his school friends in forming a resistance group. His peers saw his blindness as an asset, and he was put in charge of recruitment, screening out potential double agents:

Like the others, Georges had the idea that, being blind, I had greater faculties – tremendous ones – for seeing through people. One day George said to me, 'I must introduce you to Nivel. This character doesn't seem to be at all reliable.'

Lusseyran agreed that Nivel was untrustworthy, based on the way he spoke: 'There were lumps in the man's voice,' he said. Lusseyran and Georges were vindicated a few months later when Nivel was seen amongst the special police, wearing a Nazi badge and shouting 'Heil Hitler'.

Speaking about this skill later in life, Lusseyran talks about how the eyes can deceive: 'Think of the disastrous errors in our judgement when we base them on the clothes, the hairdo, and the smile of the person we meet.'

Lusseyran's blindness, and his revolutionary activities, didn't affect his performance at school. He went to the prestigious Lycée Louis-le-Grand, the school of Molière, Edgar Degas and Georges Pompidou, then to the elite Upper First class at the University of Paris. He should have progressed to one of the grandes écoles, but fell foul of a fascist policy introduced in 1942, prohibiting blind people from public sector employment and from attending top schools. His teachers managed to obtain an exception to this rule from the Director of Higher Education, allowing Lusseyran to take the school's entrance exams, only to have this overruled by the Minister of Education himself, Abel Bonnard. This judgement leads to one of the only flashes of anger in Lusseyran's writing, although he remains typically restrained:

I think it would be fruitless to go into the grief and anger I suffered in the hours which followed.

Like James, Lusseyran ended up in prison. After being arrested in July 1943, he was sent to the Buchenwald concentration camp, which he describes in horrific detail. He was housed in the 'invalid block', where 1,500 men lived in quarters designed for 300 people. Lusseyran describes his roommates as:

The one-legged, the one-armed, the trepanned, the deaf, the deaf-mute, the blind, the legless, the aphasic, the ataxic, the epileptic, the gangrenous, the scrofulous, the tubercular, the cancerous, the syphilitic, the old men over seventy, the boys under sixteen, the kleptomaniacs, the tramps, the perverts, and last of all the flock of madmen.

Unlike the Minister of Education, the Nazis realised that he was capable of work, and they used him as an interpreter of French, German and Russian, although he confesses in his autobiography that he didn't know a word of Russian at the time. If he had been deemed unfit for work it is unlikely he would have survived: only 30 of the 2,000 men who arrived at the camp with him were alive by the end of the war.

Lusseyran didn't continue his studies after the war. Bonnard's ruling was only overturned in 1955. Instead he taught in Greece and then in the United States. His last job was as Professor of French Literature at the University of Hawaii, and he died in 1971.

Beyond their vision loss and spending time in prison, Jacques and James don't seem to have much in common: the intellectual Parisian who became a professor, and the boy from Kent who opted out of school in his early teens. However, James and Jacques share a stoicism, a cheerfulness and a refusal to allow their poor sight to limit their activities. Lusseyran writes beautifully, but I'll end this chapter with a quotation from James, speaking about how he refuses to dwell on the injustice of his lifelong visual impairment: 'Yeah, well, there's fuck all I can do about it, innit?'

Notes

1   Farraher, Friedrichsen and Fitzgibbons, 2013.
2   Onania, 1730.
3   Laqueur, 2003.
4   *A Short Treatise on Onanism*, 1767.
5   Onanis, 1781.
6   Sorsby, 1930.
7   García Fernández, Navarro and Castaño, 2012.
8   Al Rubaie and Arevalo, 2014.
9   Friberg, Braunstein and Bressler, 1995.
10 Berne, 1964.
11 Roos, 2012.
12 Mounsey, 2015.
13 Spiers et al., 2016.
14 Torre et al., 2022.
15 Schuch and Stubbs, 2019.
16 Smith et al., 2013.
17 Nollett et al., 2016.
18 Kroenke, Spitzer and Willianms, 2003.
19 Strawbridge, Wallhagen and Shema, 2007.
20 Bertrand et al., 2022.
21 Tiller, 2013.
22 Frank et al., 2019.
23 van der Ham et al., 2021a.
24 van der Ham et al., 2021b.
25 Lee, Park and Park, 2022.
26 Smith et al., 2022.

27   Lam et al., 2008.
28   Akram and Batool, 2020.
29   Cooney et al., 2013.
30   Dunn et al., 2005.
31   Forsman et al., 2012.
32   McKenzie et al., 2013.
33   Hallgren et al., 2020.
34   Martinsen, 2008.
35   Ruiz-Comellas et al., 2022.
36   Mackay and Neill, 2010.
37   Brunes, Flanders and Augestad, 2017.
38   Jones, Murray and Gomes, 2022.
39   National Institute for Health and Care Excellence, 2022.
40   van der Aa et al., 2015.
41   Ferrey, Moore and Jolly, 2022.
42   Silverstein, Wang and Roche, 2013.
43   Leivada and Boeckx, 2014.
44   Pollak and Corlett, 2020.
45   Chevigny and Braverman, 1950.
46   Jefsen et al., 2020.
47   Lusseyran, 1963.

7
Look with thine ears: travelling and dating with vision impairment

When I did my professional qualifications in 1999, I had to comment on two objects as part of my 'management of partial sight' exam. The first was a magnifying glass. It would amaze most people to know what you can say about a simple lens: 'This is a 20 dioptre stand magnifier, giving an image magnification of five times, or a manufacturer's magnification of 6×, so it is marked with a number six. The lens is set closer to the object than the focal length, so the light emerging from the magnifier is divergent, so a presbyopic user will need to wear reading glasses with it,' and so on.

The second object was always a non-optical aid to help people with poor vision. In my case it was a plastic rectangle about the same size as a paperback book, with the word TAXI in high-contrast letters. A small notch was cut out of the top left corner. This was for people to hold up on the side of the road, to hail a taxi and advise the driver that the bearer was visually impaired. The notch showed which way up to hold the sign, to avoid the embarrassment of holding it upside down.

Twenty years later, it is inconceivable that anyone would use one of these as nearly everyone, sight impaired or not, would use their smartphone to summon a taxi. This has the added advantage of giving a perfect location, avoiding the pre-iPhone conversations along the lines of 'I'm outside the terminal … near a sign that says entrance to all flights … do you see where it says British Airways? … what colour is your car? … oh yes, I see you, yes that's me waving,' as well as removing the 'he's just turning into your road' line that minicab offices tended to give when they were phoned to ask where a booked taxi was.

Maybe the late nineties were a more innocent time, but I don't recall any stories of blind people being kidnapped by rogue minicab drivers when holding a taxi sign. Today it seems almost irresponsible to put potentially vulnerable people at the mercy of anyone with a car who cares to stop. For people with vision impairment, taxi apps like Bolt and Uber give the safety net of a quickly summoned taxi and provide a socially acceptable way to travel. The former president of the Lighthouse for the Blind in the USA has called Uber 'the single best advancement for the mobility of blind people in the past decade'.[1]

The taxi card was relatively discreet, but symbols of vision impairment like a guide dog or white cane are far more obvious and are a label that many people choose not to display.

Guide dogs

Although less than 1 per cent of people who have vision impairment have a guide dog – I probably only see one or two guide dog users each year in the low vision clinic – popular perception is that they are used by everyone with sight loss. Blind journalist and broadcaster Peter White tells an entertaining story about the umpteenth time he was asked: 'Where's your guide dog, mate,' at which point he snapped and said: 'Oh my God, I must have left it on the train!' This led to 'utter chaos' including the suspension of London Underground's Bakerloo Line, followed by White sheepishly confessing that he had never had a guide dog in his life.[2]

Guide dogs have been used for hundreds of years. A German encyclopaedia from 1491 called *Ortus Sanitatis* shows a blind man holding a dog on a lead, which is thought to be an early example of a guide dog. Although it might sound like an April Fool's joke, the Guide Horse Foundation trains miniature horses as mobility aids for people who are allergic to dogs and they claim that 27 per cent of people who responded to a poll said they would prefer a guide horse to another animal.[3]

White canes

Although slightly less obvious than a guide dog, white canes are another visible 'badge' of sight loss. In his project 'Mobility Device', artist Carmen Papalia absurdly highlights how conspicuous he feels when travelling with his white cane. Instead of using a more conventional mobility aid, he asked a high-school marching brass band to follow him around, playing different sounds to warn him of obstacles and steps (two ascending notes for a step up, a trill for an unmovable object). Although he said that it started out as a joke (at the start of the performance he casually says 'I got rid of my cane and I have my marching band …'), Papalia also comments on how his white cane separates him from people and how he feels like a 'strange kind of celebrity' when he uses a mobility device in public. After the band has followed him up and down stairs, across streets and into a small shop where he buys a bottle of Coke, Papalia says he found the band surprisingly efficient and that he felt he was walking more quickly than he would normally.[4]

Although they are conspicuous, white canes can be extremely helpful in crowded environments. I have been told more than once that a crowd of people can be 'parted like Moses parting the Red Sea' when a symbol cane is shown to them. They are such a well-known symbol of sight loss that they can reduce the risk of confrontation, making it obvious why someone has bumped into another customer in a crowded pub, for example. Someone with severe vision loss once told me he always sits in the first class carriage on trains, despite having standard class tickets. When asked to move by the ticket inspector, he graciously says: 'Oh, I'm awfully sorry, I didn't realise,' then slowly unfolds his symbol cane. He told me he was always then told to stay in the comfortable first class seat.

Mobility aids can attract unwanted attention. Some people feel more vulnerable when showing such an obvious sign of disability and others received unkind comments like 'How can you see your phone if you've got a white cane?' More often, bystanders try to unnecessarily help the cane user. Being helped across the road is so common that there is an entry in the index of David Blunkett's memoir headed 'blind people: roads, taken across'. He writes:

> Quite frequently, when I paused at a curb, someone would grab my arm and steer me across the street, lifting me bodily up the curb the other side, without so much as a by-your-leave. They did so with the best intentions, naturally, but it was irritating to find myself suddenly sailing across the road, particularly if I was actually intending to head off in another direction.[5]

For many years, researchers have tried to develop more discreet mobility aids for people with vision impairment. One option is to use a LiDAR laser scanner, which is incorporated on some high-end smartphones. This invisible laser scans the area in front of the user and will indicate the presence of obstacles by emitting a high-pitched sound, which is heard through earphones.[6] LidSonic is a system that incorporates scanners onto a pair of 'smart glasses', giving audio warnings and spoken descriptions of obstacles,[7] which sounds promising but isn't yet available commercially.

Other researchers have tried using a 'buzzing belt', which vibrates in the location that corresponds to a potential collision.[8] People with vision impairment made fewer errors when navigating an indoor maze wearing this 'LEO' belt, but walked more slowly than when they weren't using it.

One problem with developing new mobility aids is that white canes are extremely effective when they are used properly, which sets a very high bar for any new system. Even when new mobility devices sound impressive, they don't avoid every collision. A rigorous trial of one video camera-based system found a reduction in unintended 'contacts' when the device was switched on – but the users still bumped into 9 per cent of obstacles every hour.[9] If this 'contact' leads to a fall, a broken hip or even a bruised shin, it is still one 'contact' too many.

New technology: good and bad

Although technology can be a great help to people with vision impairment, some innovations make life more difficult for those who can't see well.

Perhaps the most dangerous new technology for people with sight loss is the electric car. Most people with vision impairment rely on sound to determine whether it is safe to cross a road, with some mobility instructors recommending that people wait for an 'all quiet' gap in vehicle sounds before stepping off the kerb.[10] This technique might have been appropriate in quiet neighbourhoods when cars and motorbikes were louder, but is less useful in a twenty-first-century city filled with near-silent electric cars, e-scooters, electric bikes and zero-emission buses. Deborah Kent Stein from the USA's National Federation of the Blind describes her first encounter with a hybrid car, in 2003:

> 'When are you going to start?' I asked [the friend demonstrating her Toyota Prius].
>
> 'I did start,' our friend answered. 'I drove down to the end of the block, and then I backed past you and drove up in front of you again.'
>
> I felt a cold sense of dread. I thought, we've got a real problem.[11]

Some researchers have developed vehicle detection devices that can be used by the person with vision impairment,[12] but this is an unsatisfactory approach for three reasons. First the responsibility is then shifted onto the pedestrian who can't see – the most vulnerable person in this situation – rather than the driver. Second, this relies on everyone with vision impairment carrying one of these devices, using it effectively and it working with 100 per cent accuracy. Finally, inclusive design means that making road crossing safer for people with vision impairment will improve the urban environment for everyone, from the teenager who is paying more attention to her phone than the street, to the distracted parent who is trying to supervise three children at the same time as crossing the road.

Requiring electronic cars to make a noise is the solution that has been suggested in most countries. Japan led the world in hybrid and electric cars and in regulating their sound in 2010; the European Union and United States followed a few years later. The European approach is that electric cars 'should sound similar to the sound of a vehicle of the same category equipped with an internal combustion engine'. Although some manufacturers wanted to be able to create new sounds for electric cars (including the ridiculous idea of having a flatulent Tesla),[11] most regulators have rejected any audible warning that doesn't sound like an existing vehicle.

Travelling

Mobility isn't only about getting from your home to the local shop, or commuting to work. Many people also enjoy exploring unfamiliar environments on holiday or weekends away – although not many were as adventurous as James Holman. A traveller of the Phileas Fogg style, he visited almost every country in the world and in the 1820s he travelled across Siberia in an open horse-drawn carriage taking only six bottles of brandy, six bottles of French wine, some tea leaves, a kettle and cups, and some medicines.

At a time when taking a 'grand tour' was a staple part of being an upper-class British man, Holman stands out in two respects. Firstly, he wasn't from an aristocratic family – his father was an apothecary, a solid middle-class profession. Secondly, he lost all his sight from an inflammatory eye disease in his early twenties and didn't start his adventuring until he was completely blind. Between 1819 and 1832, Holman published books describing his travels to every continent, emphasising his blindness in the titles (for example, one volume has the subtitle 'Comprising incidents that occurred to the author, who has long suffered under a total deprivation of sight').

Holman travelled ceaselessly and used a noctograph – a device invented by Ralph Wedgwood for writing at night, consisting of carbon paper and tactile guidelines – to write detailed notes about the people he met and the places he visited. He kept meticulous records of the weather. During a winter in St Petersburg, he reported four days as being: 'Snowy. Very dull. Ditto, with snow. Ditto.'

He received some unpleasant comments about travelling without sight. A former travelling companion of his reportedly complained that 'he, indeed, may go there (Siberia), as well as anywhere else, for he will see just as much; but there is so little to be seen by those who have even the use of their eyes, that I cannot divine what interest he can have to attempt it'. Holman rebutted this criticism with elegance, saying (perhaps pointedly) that as he was 'freed from the hazard of being misled by appearances, I am the less likely to adopt hasty and erroneous conclusions'.[13]

Stephen Kuusisto is a poet who is sometimes asked to justify why he should love travelling when he can't see. In his book *Eavesdropping: A Memoir of Blindness and Listening*, he answers this by writing that:

> One can hear baroque music in Venice or dine on softshell crabs in Baltimore … we hear the movements of strangers; hear their laughter; hear pennies dropped in the Hilton's fountain; the bristles of a shoeshine brush; the wings of a pigeon that has made its way indoors.[14]

Kuusisto writes what he calls 'auditory postcards' and tone poems about the places he visits. These focus on the sounds he hears, starting from his early life experiences in Helsinki ('What a thrill it was to be a sightless child in a city of sounds'). He describes the:

> pleasure of simply standing still on the street. I found that I could stop anywhere – bring to a close the walking I was doing and the thinking that went with it – and suddenly the ambient noise of the neighbourhood would open around me.[14]

Other blind travellers have written about experiencing the soundscape of a city. For example, David Blunkett writes this about a visit to Manhattan:

> It is hard to describe, but from the sound of the ships' horns reverberating off the skyscrapers on the waterfront, I could picture the skyline: the sheer height of the World Trade Center, the chasms

of streets between the towering buildings, the sheer vastness of it all.[5]

John Hull describes the opposite effect, a sense of emptiness, when looking out over Fairy Park, near Melbourne, while on holiday in Australia:

> We came to the highest point, a look-out place, and I could feel the handrail. I could sense the vast, open space, the drop at my feet. The movement of air was so different and whereas before I could hear the echoing footsteps of the running children, now it was the cries of the wheeling gulls, the noise coming from the distant brick kiln down in the valley, the patterns of the roads beneath me traced out by the passing traffic and the excited comments of the sighted people gathered along the rail next to me.[15]

Despite this experience, Hull does admit to being despondent when travelling as someone with vision impairment, writing that 'it is so difficult to remain always interested and enthusiastic when people are pointing things out and reminding me of the lovely view which one can see from this spot'.[15]

My friend Kelly Carver, whose daughter wrote about having a blind father in her university application (see Chapter 3), also writes elegantly about the sensory immersion involved in visiting a new city without sight. Here, he describes engaging other senses when visiting Florence on holiday:

> Like triangulating cell phone towers, I mark the particular sounds we pass: the music from the pizza place on Orale, the odour of tanning oil billowing from a leather shop, and the chatter at the Duomo piazza cafe terrace to orientate our position, a rough sketch backup should Julie lose her bearing. I silently confirm to myself that I'd be able to direct us back to the hotel.

Kelly found traffic noise useful when traversing the narrow alleyways of Italy, in contrast to the well-ordered wide streets he is accustomed to in Minneapolis:

> From behind, we gauge the distance of the occasional approaching car or Vespa by the level of sound echoing off the gapless line of centuries old stone and cement-faced homes, each fronted by thick

12-foot-tall doors of oak bearing plate sized iron ring knockers. When forced back onto a narrow sidewalk, a safe way to travel along develops. I take the lead, dragging my cane along the front of the curb, gauging my distance from the street. Julie eyes the way ahead, calling out obstructions, loose and missing sidewalk tiles, or an oncoming pedestrian. We make good time.

Many travellers – sighted and with poor vision – would probably benefit from stopping and standing still from time to time, listening to the sounds of a neighbourhood and sensing the echo of noise from the surroundings. As Shakespeare wrote in King Lear: 'A man may see how this world goes with no eyes. Look with thine ears.'[16]

Dating with vision impairment

As well as 'disrupting' the taxi trade and the travel industry, technology has revolutionised the world of dating. People with vision impairment are now able to look at potential partners in detail, perhaps by looking at their picture on an iPad a few centimetres away from their face, before deciding whether to go on a date with someone. Gaylen Kapperman, Professor Emeritus at Northern Illinois University, has researched the likelihood of blind people getting dates through the online dating app Tinder. He asked sighted undergraduates to set up identical Tinder profiles, with and without photos including a white cane and dark glasses. For women, there was no difference in the number of interested partners, whereas 'blind' men were slightly more likely to be chosen for dates than sighted men.[17] Although this may sound encouraging, more than one of the women were told through the site that the man 'had always wanted to have sex with a blind girl'.[18] Kapperman does not report whether any of the men received the same comments but does suggest that there may be a 'mothering' element which may account for the higher success rates of the 'blind' men on the website.

Kapperman's own experiences of being told he should have a vasectomy rather than having children were mentioned in Chapter 3, reflecting some of the findings of Marissa Slaughter's PhD thesis 'Love Is Not Blind: Eugenics, Blindness and Marriage in the United States, 1840–1940'. She writes that 'in the late-nineteenth and early-twentieth centuries, eugenicists, blindness professionals, and even other blind people believed that the best way to eliminate blindness was through the restriction of marriages between blind people'. She describes the sad story of Lucien Howe, an American ophthalmologist who went from being an altruistic young doctor who travelled to Egypt and Syria treating ophthalmia neonatorum (a serious eye infection of newborn infants), to a eugenicist who used unpleasant phrases like 'improvement of a race by selective breeding' and who lobbied to stop blind people getting married.[19,20] Sadly Howe's views were not unusual at the time; Theodore Roosevelt, the twenty-sixth President of the USA, wrote that 'I wish very much that the wrong people could be prevented entirely from breeding … feebleminded persons [should be] forbidden to leave offspring behind them'.[21]

Today people with visual impairment in the USA are still less likely to get married than those with good vision,[22] and they are also more likely to divorce, with 3.3 per cent of Americans with vision impairment getting divorced in one year, compared to 2.2 per cent of people without sight loss.[23] These data come from surveys and do not attempt to explore the reasons for this higher divorce rate, but sociologist Philip Cohen speculates that it might be due to economic stress or caring obligations.

Marriage rates are declining in many high-income countries. In England and Wales, 2021 was the first year when most children were born to parents who weren't married or in a civil partnership (to highlight how quickly this has changed, consider the fact that in 1977, the year I was born, 90 per cent of babies were born to a married woman)[24] and having sex before marriage is the norm rather than a source of shame. A large survey of teenagers in Germany found that those with vision impairment tend to be older when they have their first relationship (an average of 15 years old, compared to 14 for those with good sight) but that there was no difference in the age at which they first have sex, an event that the researchers rather charmingly call their 'sexual debut'.[25]

Research has shown that adolescents with visual impairment don't have a lack of sex education (at least in enlightened countries like the Netherlands),[26] but how can blind teenagers make dating as easy as possible? In her irreverent TV series *How This Blind Girl…*,[27] Mared Jamen's character Ceri gives some tips on going on a date: choose a location you know really well and can get around inconspicuously; get there early ('let him find you, you'll never find him'); and finally 'remove all evidence of being blind: for example, reduce text size [on your phone] and turn off VoiceOver'. In later episodes of the series, she challenges the myth that blind people are 'unsexy, sexless, asexual beings', and shows embarrassing (perhaps autobiographical) details like sending intimate pictures to the wrong person, kissing her boyfriend's brother by mistake and finally 'coming out' as visually impaired. I highly recommend this series to older teenagers with vision impairment.

Notes

1   Uber, 2022.
2   BBC 'View from the Boundary', 2022.
3   The Guide Horse Foundation, 2005.
4   Grand Central Art Center, 2013.
5   Blunkett and MacCormick, 2002.
6   Yang et al., 2017.
7   Busaeed et al., 2022.
8   Brown et al., 2019.
9   Pundlik et al., 2021.
10 Peat and Higgins, 2022.
11 Seabrook, 2022.
12 Jones, 2006.
13 Roberts, 2006.
14 Kuusisto, 2006.
15 Hull, 1990.
16 Shakespeare, 1608.
17 Kapperman et al., 2017.
18 Kapperman and Kelly, 2019.
19 Stalvey, 2014.
20 Howe, 1918.
21 Ravin and Stern, 2010.
22 Cohen, 2014.
23 Cohen, 2013.
24 Office for National Statistics, 2022.
25 Pinquart and Pfeiffer, 2012.
26 Kef and Bos, 2006.
27 BBC, *How This Blind Girl …*, 2022

8
The end of blindness?

Some of the earliest recorded medical treatments were attempts to cure blindness. Some historians think that cataracts were first treated in the late Bronze Age.[1] Couching, a surgical technique used to remove cataracts, was certainly being performed more than 2,500 years ago. It was first described in an Indian medical book in about 600 BCE and was widely used in Asia and Europe by the time of the Roman Empire.[2]

Cataract is the clouding and opacification of the lens inside the eye. As a cataract progresses, it reduces visual acuity, the ability to recognise colours and the ability to see faint details. If left untreated, it can lead to complete blindness. In couching, a needle is poked into the eye, dislodging this opaque lens and pushing it back into the vitreous chamber of the eye (Figure 8.1).

This operation was performed not only by doctors. In 1583, the early German ophthalmologist Georg Bartisch wrote:

> Nor is there any lack of old women, vagrant hags, therica sellers, tooth-pullers, ruined shopkeepers, rat and mouse catchers, knaves, tinkers, hog-butchers, hangmen, bum-bailiffs, and other wanton good for nothing vagabonds … all of whom boldly try to perform this noble cure.[3]

Couching is associated with severe complications, particularly glaucoma and infection, leading Bartisch to warn people not to 'fall into the hands of such irresponsible destroyers and murderers of eyes'.[3] The composer Johann Sebastian Bach was a particularly famous victim of couching, dying in severe pain (and total blindness) four months after his cataracts were removed by couching.[4] As well as being dangerous, it also does not

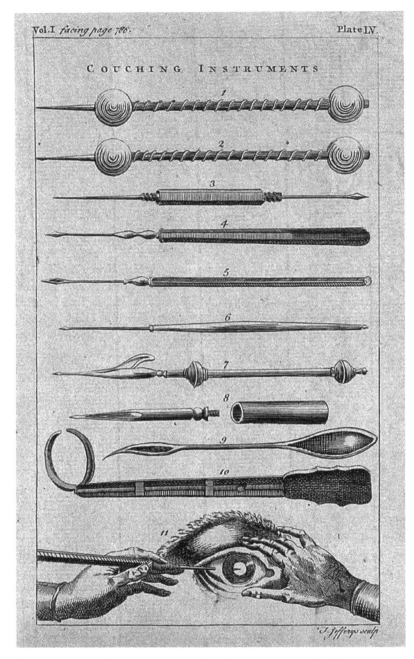

Figure 8.1 Couching instruments. Taken from an engraving by Thomas Jefferys, 1763. Source: https://creativecommons.org/use-remix/.

work very well. In 1917, a case series showed visual improvement in only 20 per cent of 550 people who had the procedure, with about 10 per cent losing all of their sight from retinal detachment.[2]

By the eighteenth century, itinerant oculists were travelling around Europe, performing couching with varying degrees of success.[5] The first 'modern' cataract operation where the lens was removed (as opposed to being prodded into the eye) was performed in France in 1752, by Jacques Daviel.[6]

After lens removal (whether by couching or Daviel's technique), the eye is left very longsighted. People without a lens in their eye tend to need glasses of about +11.00 dioptres. In some cases, this can be provided in contact lenses, but nowadays most adults who have cataract surgery have their lens replaced with a plastic intraocular lens. Lens implantation was first performed by Harold Ridley in 1949, at St Thomas's Hospital in London. It is said that after treating a Second World War pilot who had been injured by a broken plane windscreen, Ridley noticed that Perspex was quite well tolerated inside the eye, so he used a similar material as his first synthetic lens within the eye. This operation was controversial and was particularly disliked by ophthalmic surgeons at the rival Moorfields Eye Hospital in London.[7] The next big innovation in cataract surgery was the development of phacoemulsification in the 1960s. This allows microsurgical techniques to be used in cataract surgery. The cataractous lens is liquified, allowing it to be extracted through a needle, then a folded replacement lens is injected and unfolded inside the eye.[8]

Today, cataract surgery is the most commonly performed operation in the world, with tens of millions of people having safe and effective cataract operations every year.[9] By some measures, cataract surgery is thought to be the most cost-effective surgical procedure there is.[10,11]

Couching is still performed in parts of the world where there is reduced access to modern healthcare, particularly in West Africa. As well as not being particularly effective, couching is painful. Almost three-quarters of people who had experienced couching in rural Nigeria said it was painful, 87 per cent said they would not have the operation again and nearly all would now advise against couching.[12] Couching is not significantly cheaper than more effective methods of surgery. In Mali in 2010, the average cost of couching was US$42.10 and modern surgery cost US$52.40 including transport and drugs, although 'the traditional healer was often paid partially in kind and the price paid varied according to the patient's ability to pay'.[13] Even when the procedure works and the cataract is dislodged, the high-powered spectacles needed are often not available to people with limited access to modern healthcare.

Glaucoma treatment

Ophthalmology is an unusual medical specialism in that it combines surgery with medicine. Many diseases at the front of the eye, like cataract, corneal conditions and eyelid problems, are treated surgically, as are some diseases of the vitreous and retina, particularly retinal detachment. Other serious eye diseases, such as macular degeneration or retinal vein occlusions, are managed primarily with drugs. However, glaucoma is treated by a combination of drugs and surgery, making it one of the more mixed subspecialisms in ophthalmology.

Glaucoma is a progressive optic nerve disease, which is associated with an increased pressure inside the eye. Intraocular pressure is maintained by a balance of aqueous humour production and drainage of this fluid through the trabecular meshwork at the edge of the iris. If too much fluid is produced, or the fluid drains away too slowly, the pressure in the eye will rise, like a bicycle tyre being overinflated. In many people with glaucoma, this increase in intraocular pressure is the cause of their vision loss. Relatively simple drugs, like beta-blockers, can reduce the production of this fluid, while the outflow of aqueous can be increased using other drugs like latanoprost, a prostaglandin that is now the first line of treatment for many forms of glaucoma.

These drugs are usually given as eyedrops, taken once or twice per day. When used properly, eyedrops are effective at delivering drugs directly to the eye, but they do enter the circulatory system and can have side effects on other parts of the body. Beta-blocker eye drops can cause fainting, falls and even heart attacks.[14] When these drugs were more widely used as a glaucoma treatment, they were said to be the leading cause of falls in older people with glaucoma.[15] In one case report, glaucoma doctors changed a patient's medication from twice-daily beta-blockers after he collapsed in the eye clinic waiting room.[16] This man went from falling over every day to not falling once in the 10 weeks after his eye drops were changed. As the authors of this report point out, if he hadn't collapsed in the waiting room, the cause of this patient's falls might never have been identified, as people often don't think of eyedrops as drugs, often answering 'no' when asked by doctors if they take any medication.

Newer glaucoma drugs have more innocuous side effects. The most noticeable side effect of latanoprost, the first-line treatment for many forms of glaucoma,[17] is an increase in the length of the eyelashes. People often like this effect, although it can look unusual when people only use the drop in one eye and have bushier and darker eyelashes above one eye compared to the other. This side effect has been exploited by some beauticians; some 'eyelash serum' contains drugs designed to treat glaucoma, sometimes without declaring this on the label.[18] These drugs can also subtly change the colour of the iris, more noticeably in people only using the drops in one eye.

As well as side effects, a big problem with using eyedrops as a treatment is that people often don't take them – their adherence to treatment is poor. Glaucoma is a very slowly progressive condition and most people who take eyedrops to treat it will need to take them once or twice per day for their whole life. One American study found that nearly half of people with glaucoma didn't collect any more eyedrops from their pharmacy after six months, and nearly two-thirds had stopped taking their treatment after three years.[19] Similar studies from Europe have found better compliance, perhaps as there are fewer financial barriers to obtaining medication – a single bottle of latanoprost costs about £1.50 (about €1.75 or $1.90), although some American pharmacies charge from $25 (€22, £19) per bottle for a generic drug, and up to $275 (€246, £212) for a bottle of brand-name eyedrops.[20,21] However, cost isn't the only barrier to taking this medication. Even in countries with good public healthcare systems like the Netherlands, about a quarter of people with glaucoma admit to not always taking their eyedrops.[22]

Studies have shown that difficulty in putting eye drops in, poor drop technique and simple forgetfulness are barriers to using eyedrops effectively,[23,24] so many hospitals run patient education sessions where they show people how to use their drops and explain the importance of regular treatment. Devices that help people to put in their eye drops can be very helpful, as can phone apps and medication alarms to remind people to take them.

In part because of this poor adherence to drug treatment, surgery is now offered as an alternative to eyedrops in many cases.[17] A safe and painless laser operation called selective laser trabeculoplasty can be used to increase the outflow of aqueous humour from the eye. This procedure is even more effective than using eyedrops in controlling the intraocular pressure (although eyedrops are also very good: 93 per cent of people who had the operation had an ideal eye pressure after three years, compared to 91.3 per cent of those taking eyedrops).[25] Better glaucoma treatment hasn't yet led to a drop in the number of people being registered as sight impaired with this condition,[26] but the prognosis is generally good for people who have glaucoma diagnosed at an early stage, who take their eyedrops and who attend their follow-up appointments.[27,28]

Age-related macular disease

Another method of delivering drugs into the eye is to inject them directly into the vitreous humour. The development of these intravitreal drugs to treat age-related macular disease is without doubt the biggest innovation in the treatment of eye disease over my career.

When I first qualified in the late 1990s, age-related macular disease (AMD) was by far the most common cause of severe sight impairment in most high-income countries. Twenty-five years later, after the widespread adoption of injected treatments for wet AMD, the number of people over 50 years old who are blind from macular disease has fallen from 0.2 per cent to 0.1 per cent of the population.[29]

AMD can progress in two ways. The more common 'dry' type of the disease is caused by a slowly progressing atrophy of the photoreceptors in the macula. The reasons for this cell death are complex but are thought to include failure of the retinal pigment epithelium layer of the retina, with oxidative stress being a significant contributory factor.[30,31] Over time, a blind spot appears in the central part of the visual field, reducing the ability to read, to recognise faces and to see fine details. People with this condition often develop a technique called eccentric viewing, moving their eyes slightly to one side of what they want to look at, 'catching' the image with healthy retina just outside their damaged macula.[32,33] Back in the 1990s, it was common to hear people with dry age-related macular disease being told they were 'lucky' or 'had the good type', as this form of the condition progressed more slowly and tended not to affect the vision as much as the quicker, 'wet' form of this disease where vision can be lost almost overnight. In wet AMD, new blood vessels grow under or into the macula, where they can leak fluid, leading to distorted vision and a rapidly progressing blind spot. This neovascular process is stimulated, in part, by the expression of a protein called vascular endothelial growth factor (VEGF). This protein is produced in response to a lack of oxygen and has been implicated in many diseases including asthma,[34] some cancers,[35] inflammatory bowel disease[36] and COVID-19,[37] as well as in retinal disease.

Drugs that inhibit VEGF, such as ranibizumab, aflibercept, brolucizumab, faricimab and bevacizumab, are known as anti-angiogenic or anti-VEGF agents. A tiny quantity of this drug (typically about 0.2 millilitres) is injected through the white of the eye while the patient looks in the opposite direction. Although many people dislike the thought of having an injection into the eye, the Macular Society reassures their members that these injections are 'much less frightening than they sound',[38] which matches my experience. People who have had these injections usually tell me it is a quick and painless procedure, similar to visiting the dentist. In one study of people who had been receiving intravitreal injections for one year, almost half agreed with the statement 'I am afraid of the treatment,' (one-third thought 'the number of ophthalmological visits is arduous'), but over 90 per cent said that they would choose the treatment again.[39] Anti-angiogenic drugs are nearly always given as a series of injections. On average, people receive seven injections in the first year of treatment,[40] often with a 'loading phase' of one injection per month for three months, followed by injections when there is any sign of recurrence of the disease.

The first randomised controlled trial of an anti-angiogenic drug for wet AMD was published in 2006 and is already one of the most cited papers in the history of ophthalmology.[41,42] Since this paper was published, hundreds of thousands of doses of these drugs have been injected, with many eye hospitals building new treatment suites for the delivery of intravitreal injections. The most recent national audit in the UK showed that the disease was stabilised in 90 per cent of those who received treatment, with significant vision improvement in 20 per cent.[40] These drugs are also used for people with other types of retinal disease, such as retinal vein occlusion,[43] diabetic eye disease[44] and maculopathy associated with high myopia.[45]

The success of these treatments means that over the last few years, dry AMD has come to be seen as the 'unlucky' form to have. The search for an effective treatment for dry age-related macular degeneration is being funded by many charities, funding bodies and drug companies around the world, and it seems likely that medical treatment for this condition will emerge soon. Indeed, as I finished this chapter, I learned that pegcetacoplan, known as Syfovre, had been licensed by the Food and Drug Administration in the USA for the treatment of dry macular disease. In a randomised controlled trial, this drug, which is injected into the eye every one or two months, reduced the progression of dry AMD, but did not restore vision.[46] It remains to be seen whether this drug will revolutionise the treatment of macular disease (and earn billions of dollars for the drug company) as did intravitreal injections for wet AMD.

Stem cell therapy

Another avenue of research for the treatment of dry AMD is to use stem cells. Human stem cells are undifferentiated cells that can develop into various different types of cell and can proliferate indefinitely. Some stem cells, such as those found in a human embryo, are pluripotent – that is, they can form into almost any structure in the body. This makes them a very tempting way to treat disease – if human embryonic stem cells are implanted into the retina, can they form new retinal cells to replace those that have been damaged by macular degeneration?

Implanting human cells into the body, ensuring that they are not rejected by the recipient and making them differentiate into the correct type of retinal cell is phenomenally complicated and requires interactions between surgeons, cell biologists, neuroscientists, ophthalmologists, pharmacologists, virologists and even ethicists – there are huge moral considerations when implanting cells derived from a human embryo into an unrelated adult.[47] Despite this complexity, there is some early evidence that this might be a viable treatment for some people with retinal disease.[48–52] It will be interesting to see whether stem cell therapy or medication becomes the standard treatment for dry macular degeneration over the next decade or so.

New therapies for rare diseases

It isn't only common diseases like age-related macular disease that are treated with new drugs. For example, Leber Hereditary Optic Neuropathy (LHON) is a very rare disease which affects only about one in 50,000 people, usually young men.[53] LHON has a particularly large impact on visual function, with one study suggesting that it reduces vision-related quality of life more than any other eye disease.[54] Some people with LHON respond well to a drug called idebenone, a compound that is related to co-enzyme Q_{10}. It is difficult to assess quite how useful idebenone is – LHON is a rare disease, there are different forms of the condition caused by different genes and some people with LHON have a spontaneous improvement in vision without taking any therapy – but it seems that there is a significant benefit to taking this treatment.[55] I have seen people in the low vision clinic who have experienced remarkable changes in their vision after taking idebedone. I think it is particularly encouraging to people with rare diseases that drug companies aren't only interested in developing the next 'blockbuster' drug for very common conditions like dry AMD.

Gene therapy

It is impossible to write anything about medical treatment in the twenty-first century without acknowledging the staggering recent progress in genetic research. It took 13 years and three billion dollars to map the first human genome, which was completed in 2003. Today, the whole genome can be sequenced in days for a few hundred dollars, and this time and cost is falling rapidly. The National Health Service in the UK aims to be the world's first national health care system to offer whole genome sequencing as part of routine care. It is on the way to sampling hundreds of thousands of complete genomes as part of the Biobank study.[56] Genomic sequencing is a phenomenal achievement which has been made possible by technological advances in many areas, not least in data storage. Even stored as a compressed zip file, a complete human genome takes up a huge amount of computer memory.[57]

One consequence of these advances in genetics is that diseases are often now defined by their genetic basis instead of their symptoms or how they look in the eye. It is now more common for me to hear a diagnosis of 'ABCA4 retinopathy' or 'CRB1 degenerative retinal disease' than a term like 'Stargardt disease' or 'retinitis pigmentosa'. Conditions that were previously thought of as one disease, or perhaps as following one type of inheritance pattern (such as autosomal dominant optic atrophy) are now described by the exact gene that is affected. Knowing the genotype of a disease improves the prediction of the onset, severity, prognosis and treatment potential of the disease. It also opens up the possibility of replacing that gene with a healthier copy, which is the principle of gene therapy.

Eye diseases are not serious enough to warrant pre-implantation genetic testing, where the embryo implanted in an in-vitro fertilisation procedure is selected to exclude those with the disease, which is more widely used for potentially fatal conditions like Tay-Sach's disease.[58] Instead, gene therapy in ophthalmology is performed after birth, most commonly on teenagers or adults with severe inherited retinal disease.

The first trials of human gene therapy for eye disease were for retinal degenerations caused by the RPE65 gene, and involved complementary DNA being combined with a virus (to enable it to enter individual cells) and injected into the eye. The first results from two competing groups – in London and in Pennsylvania – were announced at the biggest eye research meeting in the world in May 2008, and published alongside each other in the *New England Journal of Medicine*.

These early trials were designed to assess the safety and feasibility of the treatment and not to determine its effect, although the London team reported that 'one patient [of three] had a significant improvement in visual function'[59] and the US group, who also treated three young adults, said that 'each patient had a modest improvement in measures of retinal function on subjective tests'.[60] This treatment is now available clinically as voretigene neparvovec (Luxturna) and has shown to improve visual fields, sensitivity to light and performance on a mobility task, especially in dim light. Despite its very high cost (the cost of the gene therapy agent alone is over £600,000)[61] and relatively modest effect on visual function, this treatment has been approved by regulators in the UK, EU, Canada and Australia. It was the first ever in vivo gene therapy licensed for human disease by the Food and Drug Administration in the USA.

Other diseases for which gene therapy is being developed include other forms of retinal degeneration (including those caused by RHO, USH2A and RPGR),[62] choroideremia (CHM),[63] Stargardt disease (ABCA4)[64] and wet age-related macular degeneration.[65]

Gene therapy has also been used for a very rare inherited retinal disease called achromatopsia.[66] Unlike some other inherited retinal diseases, people with achromatopsia have vision impairment from birth – they have a very serious malfunction of their retinal cone cells. This causes their visual system to be reliant on rod photoreceptors, the cells that are usually used primarily for dark-adapted vision. In daylight, people with achromatopsia have extreme sensitivity to light, reduced visual acuity and an absence of colour vision. Unlike most people with 'colour blindness', who still perceive colours but confuse some colours with each other, people with achromatopsia really see the world as it would appear on a black and white television.

Treating achromatopsia with gene therapy raises some fascinating scientific questions, touched on in Chapter 4 of this book. Can the brain respond to new inputs from cone cells if it has developed without using these signals at all? Can people see colour when they didn't see it as a child? Colleagues of mine in the Child Vision Lab at UCL are attempting to answer these questions using a combination of brain imaging and psychophysical experiments. They have shown new cone-mediated activity in some children who have received this treatment and report that, in some people, gene therapy can indeed 'evoke visual signals not previously experienced'.[67]

The impact of treatment for eye disease – from remarkable blind person to average sighted person

Not all optometrists work with blind people. Most work on high streets or in shopping centres, prescribing spectacles and contact lenses to people without serious sight problems. Others, like my friend Jenni, specialise in other niches. Jenni is fascinated by changes in shape of the cornea, the clear front surface of the eye, through which light is focused. The eye is so complex that Jenni's interest extends only to that tiny structure, half a millimetre thick, so if her patients have a problem with part of the eye just a few microns away she will refer them to a colleague who deals with that structure.

I've always assumed that Jenni's interest in the cornea is linked to her passion for photography. I remember once showing her a second-hand Russian SLR camera that I'd found in my father-in-law's house. I loved it as the Cyrillic script reminded me of Cold War films, but Jenni was less keen. 'It's fine,' she said, 'but I couldn't use that lens. I'm so used to looking through high-quality optics.'

Like my battered Soviet camera, the cornea's performance is degraded by tiny imperfections. Changes in curvature of a fraction of a millimetre can distort the vision so much that it renders someone blind, while a corneal scar the size of a pinpoint can scatter light so much that the glare makes going outside without sunglasses unbearable.

To help her patients, Jenni first makes a mould of the cornea, using a silicone liquid held in front of the eye in a small basket. She uses this mould to make a contact lens that exactly matches the profile of the patient's cornea, in effect smoothing out the imperfections in its shape. This can have dramatic visual effects. It is not uncommon for Jenni's patients to go from reading only the top letter of the chart to reading the bottom line perfectly as soon as she puts the bespoke lens on the front of their eye.

Jenni's work rarely has such a profound effect as it did on Gemma. Gemma had been born with only one working eye. Her other eye was small and its optic nerve was not fully formed. As a teenager she developed keratoconus in her 'good' eye, a condition where the cornea becomes thinner, steeper and distorted. I was taught that the shape of the cornea in keratoconus is the same as someone pointing their finger through from the inside of an inflated balloon, i.e. the regular curved surface is disrupted by an unexpected sharp point.

Jenni told me about the effect of fitting a bespoke contact lens in Gemma's eye:

I told her that I could probably fix the keratoconic eye, distorted corneas were definitely my speciality. But here we were with her registered blind with a guide dog. How would this pan out? I proceeded to fit a scleral lens to see if I could improve her vision, taking care to manage her expectations with sensitivity. We had success and achieved far better than expected. Good enough standard of vision to drive!

Jenni didn't need to be a specialist in low vision to realise the implications of this. She had restored sight in someone who very much identified as a vision-impaired woman. Gemma was a piano tuner, a common 'blind' occupation, and her partner only knew her as a blind person. Would she have to relinquish her certificate of visual impairment? Would she need to return her guide dog?

A week later, Jenni spoke to Gemma again:

She phoned me the next week in a very excited tone and explained that she was able to see well and tolerated her lens far better than she expected. She had been able to cycle again – she had not done for years. I was pleased and worried at the same time. I had never had to consider the functional and social implications of suddenly seeing clearly after years in a blur.

Gemma's life changed in many ways when Jenni restored her sight. Her driving licence was reinstated and her guide dog was retired. She also broke up with her partner and moved to a different city, events that may or may not be linked to her change in visual status, moving back from Stephen Kuusisto's 'planet of the blind' to the visually dominated world.

Gemma's experience is unusual but not unprecedented. Mike May is a larger-than-life character who is a passionate advocate for blind people and a former president of the San Francisco LightHouse for the Blind and Visually Impaired. His most famous anecdote is about skiing at the 1984 Winter Olympics. Despite being completely blind and not having permission to be anywhere near the Olympic slope, he managed not only to ski down the slope but also to be recorded descending at 65 miles per hour. The full story begins with some shaky press accreditation and ends with him being confronted by armed Yugoslavian guards. Mike is a skilled storyteller and is much in demand as a motivational speaker.

He was blinded at the age of three by a chemical explosion, causing his corneas to opacify, reducing his sight. After several unsuccessful operations, at the age of 43 he was offered revolutionary new surgery.

First, stem cells were transplanted to the edge of his cornea, followed later by a transplant of the whole cornea. Mike had received corneal transplants before, but they had always failed, usually as the cornea was rejected by his body. These operations worked and Mike's vision was restored, with one significant drawback. Mike had gone blind at the age of three, so his visual system was only as developed as that of a toddler. He was a middle-aged man with the vision of a three-year-old.

Mike's biography describes the days immediately following his surgery. His vision had a child's innocence. He did not fall for visual illusions, he was particularly interested in colour and corporate logos, and his wife had to tell him to stop staring at women in the street. In a moving passage, May describes being moved almost to tears by seeing someone sleeping rough in San Francisco. By the age of five, my daughter was sadly accustomed to seeing homeless people on the streets of London, but I still remember her shock when she first saw people sleeping on the street. It is a sad reflection of our society that we lose this sense of upset when seeing such a common urban experience.

An interesting element of Mike's vision restoration is how things that were previously remarkable became mundane. As an American, his peers perceived a blind man being able to catch a bus in Europe as miraculous. As someone with sight, it was so ordinary as to be boring. His status changed overnight, from a blind superhero to an average man in the street. This transition could be as profound as the transition from having good vision to going blind.[68]

Like Jenni, Mike May's doctors knew the risks of suddenly restoring someone's sight. In the 1960s, we didn't know what effect this would have. Known as 'the man who was disappointed by what he saw', Sidney Bradford was a blind man who had his sight restored in the middle of the twentieth century. He was studied extensively by psychologist Richard Gregory. Here Gregory describes how he first learned about the man who became his most famous subject:

> It was my research assistant, Jean Wallace, who saw in a local paper in 1959 that a man, blind from birth and now 52, was about to receive new eyes – or rather, corneal grafts that might allow him to see. We gathered up every visual trick and gadget we thought might be relevant from the practical class we ran in the Cambridge Psychological Laboratory. Dropping teaching and other commitments, we drove to a Midlands hospital in time to see Bradford just after his first eye was opened to the light.[69]

Sidney Bradford was exposed to multiple sight tests from the moment he opened his eyes. Immediately after his bandages were removed, Bradford was asked to try to tell the time on clocks, and even after leaving hospital, Gregory and his team spent a lot of time with him. It wasn't Sidney's family who first took him to the zoo to see if he could recognise an elephant – it was Richard Gregory.

Gregory didn't immediately warm to his patient, saying: 'He was just an ordinary, very sort of taciturn, Midlands, English chap. There was nothing special about him at all really, he had a rather limited sense of humour ... .'[70]

Despite this slow beginning, it is clear from Gregory's monographs that the two men became fond of one another. A few weeks after the operation, Gregory showed him around London, with disappointing results:

> We took him round London, and showed him several of the 'sights', but he was almost uniformly bored. He found all buildings dull, of no interest. His only signs of appreciation were to moving objects, particularly the pigeons in Trafalgar Square. He took great interest in them and liked to touch them while he watched. He described how as a blind man he often felt isolated and sought sounds of activity and movement.[71]

More successful was a trip to London Zoo. Gregory writes:

> He was amused by the elephants and giraffes, and particularly amused when he saw two giraffe heads looking at him from high up over the top of an adjacent cage. This was the only visual situation noted which ever made him laugh. He was allowed to throw cabbages into the mouths of the hippopotamus and his aim was good.[71]

Gregory did very well out of Bradford's case. As well as publishing several papers and monographs describing Bradford, Gregory gave the 1967 Royal Institution Christmas Lectures, his *Oxford Companion to the Mind* is still a staple of middle-class bookshelves, and in 1993 he received the ultimate accolade of being featured on BBC Radio 4's *Desert Island Discs*.

Sidney Bradford did less well and became very depressed. A year after the operation, Gregory wrote:

> He certainly relied a great deal on vision, but we formed the impression that this very reliance cost him his self-respect, for he

had been proud of his abilities when the handicap was obvious, but now his previous achievements seemed paltry and his present position almost foolish. He was not a man to talk freely, but was obviously depressed, and we felt that he had lost more than he had gained by recovery of sight …

When his handicap was apparently swept away, as by a miracle, he lost his peace and his self-respect. We may feel disappointment at a private dream come true: S.B. found disappointment with what he took to be reality.[71]

Sidney Bradford died on 2 August 1960, the year after his operation. Speaking in 2010, shortly before his own death, Richard Gregory sounds upset by the depression which Bradford experienced: 'I don't think those of us who tried to look after him realised what a traumatic situation it was for him, so I think to some extent we were to blame for this.'[70]

Artificial intelligence – here to save the day?

If gene therapy is one defining scientific breakthrough of the twenty-first century so far, artificial intelligence (AI) must be the other, and it has already been adopted in ophthalmology. Hundreds of thousands of retinal scans have been used to train AI systems to identify eye disease[72,73] by researchers working alongside tech giants like Google. In one study, a deep learning strategy trained an algorithm to make a decision on whether or not to refer a patient for treatment. After learning from 14,884 scans, a task that would take a human thousands of hours, the algorithm could make these referrals with the same accuracy as expert ophthalmologists and optometrists.[74] Clinicians seem happy to accept this technology, with 88 per cent of respondents to one survey of over 1,100 ophthalmologists indicating that they would be willing to use AI-based assistive tools for decision making or diagnosis,[75] particularly for diabetic retinopathy screening (a task currently performed manually, usually by an expert observing a retinal photograph on a computer screen). The ophthalmologists did not seem particularly threatened by the technology; two-thirds were confident that they will not be replaced by an algorithm,[75] although this might be overconfident given the likely emergence of autonomous robots to perform eye surgery.[76,77]

Artificial intelligence is already helping people who have vision impairment every day. Seeing AI is a suite of applications, designed by

Microsoft, which can be downloaded free of charge to iPhones and iPads. This application uses artificial intelligence to read text out loud from whatever is shown in front of the camera, making it useful for seeing signs, reading menus or even handwritten notes, with reasonable accuracy.[78] When I demonstrate Seeing AI in clinic, people are usually most interested in the face-identification mode, as they are often upset by walking past their friends in the street without recognising them. When trained on a couple of photos, Seeing AI is able to identify faces relatively well ('Michael Crossland is in front of you'). If the face isn't recognised by the app, it makes an estimate of the age, gender and expression, and is often uncannily accurate ('a 41-year-old woman with brown hair looking happy'). I suspect that a high proportion of people who use Seeing AI end up checking the apparent age of their friends in the pub within a few days of downloading it.

Seeing AI will also perform the more complex task of identifying a scene and reading a description of it aloud. Sometimes this is very impressive, but at other times it is almost laughably inaccurate. Figure 8.2 shows two images, taken on the same day. One image is described correctly as 'probably a little girl brushing her teeth with a toothbrush in his mouth' (a description that does the immensely difficult task of identifying the scene but fails at the far simpler task of matching the pronouns), but the other, of a kettle on a hob, is incorrectly tagged as 'probably a cat sitting on a counter'. My cat was lucky that I knew this

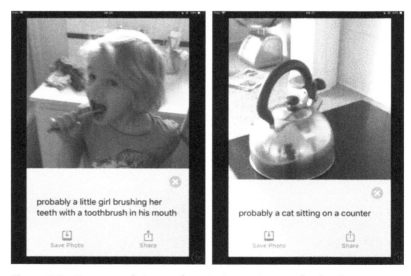

Figure 8.2 Two example images from Seeing AI. See text for details. Image: Author's own.

wasn't the case, but even on close inspection of the image, it's difficult to see what feature of the kettle looked anything like an animal.

Currently, Seeing AI and similar apps run on a smartphone, which needs to be held in front of the user to generate the description. An alternative approach is used by the OrCam MyEye, a hands-free device that does many of the same tasks from a small unit, about the size of a thumb, mounted on the side of a pair of glasses. This is less obtrusive, particularly for someone with long hair who can hide part of the unit, although it is far more expensive than a smartphone. OrCam improves some aspects of quality of life in people with vision impairment,[79] although in a recent study comparing Seeing AI to OrCam, text reading ability was about the same.[80]

Google suggests their Lookout app, which is similar to Seeing AI, is used when the phone is in a shirt pocket, with the camera peeking out. This is less obvious than holding a smartphone at arm's length, but I think these systems will be most effective once smartglasses are developed and widely adopted. It is easy to imagine a system that will give a continuous commentary on the scene ahead ('The London Review Bookshop is on your right in 100 metres. The Museum Tavern is on your right in 400 metres. Your friend Priya is walking towards you') on a wearable device.

A wearable low vision aid that looks like a conventional pair of glasses, has a long battery life, provides magnification and is able to read text aloud is the dream device for people working in low vision clinics. In the 1980s, scientists at NASA and Johns Hopkins University started developing the LVES (pronounced 'Elvis'), a head-mounted system including a camera and two small television screens, one in front of each eye.[81] These television screens were small by 1980s standards, but the whole device still weighed about a kilogram, worked only in black and white and the wearer looked a little as if they had a bicycle helmet on the wrong way round, covering their eyes instead of the back of their head. LVES was not a commercial success, but dozens of wearable electronic low vision aids have been offered since then, with each generation being a little smaller and lighter.[82] These newer devices offer very impressive improvements in visual acuity and contrast sensitivity but are limited by many of the same problems which LVES' developers experienced. We showed a newer-generation wearable device to 60 people in the low vision clinic and although nearly all achieved dramatic gains in visual acuity (reading six lines more on a test chart, on average), less than half of these people said they'd actually want to use it; people said it was too heavy and looked unusual, plus they didn't like that it couldn't be worn when walking around (because it would affect their balance).[83] When he showed several older people with macular degeneration some different wearable low vision aids, my colleague Andrew Miller heard some great comments: 'it's like something out of *Star Wars*' was my favourite.

The design of low vision devices often lags behind consumer technology. I've mentioned that most teenagers I meet are now happy to use their smartphone to take a picture and magnify a sign which they can't otherwise read, but few would use an electronic low vision aid designed to do the same thing; their phone will probably have longer battery life, a brighter screen and a better camera but more importantly, nobody will look twice at a teenager using their phone. An iPad is a more cosmetically acceptable way to read the newspaper than a desktop electronic magnifier that looks like a microfiche reader. Once wearable goggles developed by Google, Meta, Microsoft or Apple enter mainstream use, then I am sure people with vision impairment will adopt them in large numbers, meaning that real-time AI-based assistance will become a reality for people with vision impairment.

The end of blindness?

AI diagnosis, new drugs, gene therapy and robotic surgeons may reduce the number of blind people in high-income countries, but it seems unlikely that these answers will help the tens of millions of people with vision impairment in the Global South. Many of the most important methods to reduce blindness are simple – universal access to clean water, good sanitation, diabetes treatment, optometrists and ophthalmologists would reduce the incidence of sight loss by millions. Even in countries with the most advanced medical systems, treatment of cortical vision impairment, related to brain damage before or at birth, remains many years away.

Focusing on treatment for eye disease presents blindness as a 'problem' to be solved and falls into the medical model of disability, where all the difficulties experienced by someone with vision impairment are related to their disease. I am much more convinced by the social model of disability, where the function of someone with vision impairment is limited by societal problems and systemic barriers.[84] Rather than a world without blindness due to the triumphs of medicine, my utopian future is of a world where people with vision impairment – or any form of disability – are free of barriers to participate fully in society and where their diversity of experience is acknowledged.

A world with no blindness wouldn't have the poetry of Stephen Kuusisto or William Blake, the art of Luka Kille or Carmen Papalia, the philosophy of John Hull or some of the comedy of Sue Townsend. Mike May and Sidney Bradford show us that life after blindness isn't necessarily better than not seeing. All these stories, along with millions of others, remind us that living with vision impairment can be just as rich and rewarding as life with 20/20 vision.

Notes

1 Leffler et al., 2020.
2 Chan, 2010.
3 Rosen, 1942.
4 Tarkkanen, 2013.
5 Leffler et al., 2021.
6 Grzybowski, Claoué and Schwartz, 2023.
7 Sarwar and Modi, 2014.
8 Kelman, 1967.
9 Venkatesh et al., 2016.
10 Agarwal and Kumar, 2011.
11 Flessa, 2022.
12 Isawumi, Kolawole and Hassan, 2013.
13 Schémann, Bakayoko and Coulibaly, 2000.
14 Nelson et al., 1986.
15 Glynn, 1991.
16 Spratt et al., 2006.
17 National Institute for Health and Care Excellence, Glaucoma, 2022.
18 Rahman et al., 2022.
19 Nordstrom et al., 2005.
20 Drugs.com, Latanoprost, accessed 31 January 2023.
21 Drugs.com, Xalatan, accessed 31 January 2023.
22 Olthoff et al., 2009.
23 Newman-Casey et al., 2015.
24 Sleath et al., 2012.
25 Gazzard et al., 2019.
26 Rahman et al., 2020.
27 Chen, 2003.
28 Johnson, 2003.
29 Jonas et al., 2017.
30 Boyer et al., 2017.
31 Beatty et al., 2000.
32 Fletcher and Schuchard, 1997.
33 Crossland et al., 2005.
34 Pałgan and Bartuzi, 2015.
35 Carmeliet, 2005.
36 Kanazawa et al., 2001.
37 Polidoro et al., 2020.
38 Macular Society, 2022.
39 Kellner et al., 2021.
40 Norridge et al., 2023.
41 Rosenfeld et al., 2006.
42 Grzybowski, 2021.
43 Schmidt-Erfurth et al., 2019.
44 Amoaku et al., 2020.
45 Cheung et al., 2017.
46 Liao et al., 2002.

47 King and Perrin, 2014.
48 Shim et al., 2017.
49 Nommiste et al., 2017.
50 da Cruz et al., 2018.
51 Jin et al., 2019.
52 Voisin et al., 2023.
53 Puomila et al., 2007.
54 Kirkman et al., 2009.
55 Chen, Yu-Wai-Man and Newman, 2022.
56 NHS Genomic Medicine Service, accessed 31 January 2023.
57 Browning and Browning, 2023.
58 Takeuchi, 2021.
59 Bainbridge et al., 2008.
60 Maguire et al., 2008.
61 National Institute for Health and Care Excellence, 2019.
62 O'Hare et al., 2021.
63 MacLaren et al., 2014.
64 Tanna et al., 2017.
65 Guimaraes et al., 2021.
66 Fischer et al., 2020.
67 Farahbakhsh, 2022.
68 Kurson, 2007.
69 Gregory, 2004.
70 Burgess, 2010.
71 Gregory and Wallace, 1963.
72 Li et al., 2019.
73 Fu et al., 2021.
74 De Fauw et al., 2018.
75 Gunasekeran et al., 2022.
76 Keller et al., 2020.
77 Alafaleq, 2023.
78 Neat et al., 2019.
79 Nguyen et al., 2022.
80 Granquist et al., 2021.
81 Massof and Rickman, 1992.
82 Deemer et al., 2018.
83 Crossland et al., 2019.
84 Marks, 1997.

Epilogue

I love working in the low vision clinic, but it can be emotionally demanding. My preferred way of decompressing after a busy clinic is my weekly lunch in a 'greasy spoon' café with my colleague Hannah Dunbar. I have worked with Hannah for years; I co-supervised her PhD on vision impairment in diabetes and we both try to balance an academic and clinical career. One thing that we often talk about is how London has changed, along with the patients we see. Compared to 20 years ago, fewer people wear regimental ties, more speak English as a second or third language, and people don't tend to swear so much. More of the people I meet in clinic have genetic disease and fewer have vision impairment from diabetes. The range of stories I hear in clinic has expanded, so in an afternoon I might meet a Greek journalist, followed by a precariously employed English builder, then a German academic. This range of backgrounds is what makes London such an amazing city. To quote Roy Porter, the city is 'a cluster of communities, great and small, famous and unsung; a city of contrasts, a congregation of diversity'.[1]

Recently, over lunch, Hannah and I were sharing stories of a difficult morning. I had been in a heavily overbooked low vision clinic and she had been breaking bad news in the genetics clinic. The conversation moved away from work to chatting about buying Christmas presents for children – her nephew is the same age as my daughter – and what we were each doing at the weekend. As we got up to walk back to the hospital, Hannah brought the conversation back to the clinic. 'Do you know what, though, Mike?' she asked me. 'Don't you just love doing a job where you can be nosy about so many different people's lives?'

I am thankful to everyone I have met in the clinic, who allow me to nose into their lives in exchange for their appointment. It feels like an uneven balance. I provide spectacles, advice and magnifiers, and they give me stories and recommendations that I pass on to other people with visual impairment. I hope this book is partial repayment for my nosiness.

Note

1   Porter, 2000.

Bibliography

'5 music videos from the '80s that prove it was the era of uncomfortable feels'. *Mic*. Accessed 30 March 2022. https://www.mic.com/articles/134415/5-music-videos-from-the-80s-that-prove-it-was-the-era-of-uncomfortable-feels.

'99% Invisible', Episode 10: 99% Sound and Feel, 2010.

A Short Treatise on Onanism. London: Fletcher and Co., 1767.

Abang, T. B. 'Blindism: Likely Causes and Preventive Measures', *Journal of Visual Impairment & Blindness* 79 (9), (1985): 400–1. https://doi.org/10.1177/0145482X8507900904.

Adelson, J. D.; Bourne, R. R. A.; Briant P. S.; Flaxman S.; Taylor, H. R.; Jonas J. B.; Amir Abdoli, A.; Woldu, A. A. et al. 'Causes of Blindness and Vision Impairment in 2020 and Trends over 30 Years, and Prevalence of Avoidable Blindness in Relation to VISION 2020: The Right to Sight: An Analysis for the Global Burden of Disease Study', *The Lancet Global Health* 9 (2), (2021): e144–60. https://doi.org/10.1016/S2214-109X(20)30489-7.

Agarwal, A.; Kumar, D. A. 'Cost-Effectiveness of Cataract Surgery', *Current Opinion in Ophthalmology* 22 (1), (2011): 15–18. https://doi.org/10.1097/ICU.0b013e3283414f64.

Akram, B.; Batool, M. 'Suicidal Behavior among the Youth with and without Sensory Impairment: Prevalence and Comparison', *OMEGA – Journal of Death and Dying* 81 (3), (2020): 393–403. https://doi.org/10.1177/0030222818779711.

Al Rubaie, K.; Arevalo, J. F. 'Valsalva Retinopathy Associated with Sexual Activity', *Case Reports in Medicine* vol. 2014, (2014): 524286. https://doi.org/10.1155/2014/524286.

Alafaleq, M. 'Robotics and Cybersurgery in Ophthalmology: A Current Perspective', *Journal of Robotic Surgery* 17, (2023): 1159–70. https://doi.org/10.1007/s11701-023-01532-y.

Amoaku, W. M.; Ghanchi, F.; Bailey, C.; Banerjee, S.; Banerjee, S.; Downey, L.; Gale, R. et al. 'Diabetic Retinopathy and Diabetic Macular Oedema Pathways and Management: UK Consensus Working Group', *Eye* 34 (Suppl 1), (2020): 1–51. https://doi.org/10.1038/s41433-020-0961-6.

Anderson, C. 'The Wales House, Longtime Lodging House for UMN Guests, Closes'. *The Minnesota Daily*. Accessed 6 September 2022. https://mndaily.com/233682/news/ctwales.

Bainbridge, J. W. B.; Smith, A. J.; Barker, S. S.; Robbie, S.; Henderson, R.; Balaggan, K.; Viswanathan, A. et al. 'Effect of Gene Therapy on Visual Function in Leber's Congenital Amaurosis', *New England Journal of Medicine* 358 (21), (2008): 2231–39. https://doi.org/10.1056/NEJMoa0802268.

Bashinsky, A. L. 'Retinopathy of Prematurity', *North Carolina Medical Journal* 78 (2), (2017): 124–28. https://doi.org/10.18043/ncm.78.2.124.

Battal, C.; Occelli, V.; Bertonati, G.; Falagiarda, F.; Collignon, O. 'General Enhancement of Spatial Hearing in Congenitally Blind People', *Psychological Science* 31 (9), (2020): 1129–39. https://doi.org/10.1177/0956797620935584.

Beatty, S.; Koh, H.-H.; Phil, M.; Henson, D.; Boulton, M. 'The Role of Oxidative Stress in the Pathogenesis of Age-Related Macular Degeneration', *Survey of Ophthalmology* 45 (2), (2000): 115–34. https://doi.org/10.1016/S0039-6257(00)00140-5.

Bendas, J.; Hummel, T.; Croy, I. 'Olfactory Function Relates to Sexual Experience in Adults', *Archives of Sexual Behavior* 47 (5), (2018): 1333–39. https://doi.org/10.1007/s10508-018-1203-x.

Berne, E. *Games People Play: The Psychology of Human Relationships*. London: Penguin, 1964.

Bertrand, R.; Vrkljan, B.; Kühne, N.; Charvoz, L.; Fournier, J.; Masse, M.; Veyre, A.; Vuillerme, N. 'When One Partner Can No Longer See: Exploring the Lived Experiences of Romantic Partners in the Context of Vision Loss', *British Journal of Visual Impairment*, (2022). https://doi.org/10.1177/02646196221139780.

Best, J.; Liu, P. Y.; Ffytche, D.; Potts, J.; Moosajee, M. 'Think Sight Loss, Think Charles Bonnet Syndrome', *Therapeutic Advances in Ophthalmology* 11 (2019): 2515841419895909. https://doi.org/10.1177/2515841419895909.

Bharwani, S. K.; Green, B. F.; Pezzullo, J. C.; Bharwani, S. S.; Bharwani, S. S.; Dhanireddy, R. 'Systematic Review and Meta-Analysis of Human Milk Intake and Retinopathy of Prematurity: A Significant Update', *Journal of Perinatology* 36 (11), (2016): 913–20. https://doi.org/10.1038/jp.2016.98.

Blunkett, D.; MacCormick. A. *On a Clear Day*, Revised edition. London: Michael O'Mara, 2002.

Bonne, N. 'Tactile Universe. Meet the Team: Nic Bonne (Project Lead)'. 2018. Accessed 15 June 2022. https://tactileuniverse.org/2018/09/17/meet-the-team-nic-bonne-project-lead.

Bowen, M.; Zutshi, H.; Cordiner, M.; Crutch, S.; Shakespeare, T. 'Qualitative, Exploratory Pilot Study to Investigate How People Living with Posterior Cortical Atrophy, Their Carers and Clinicians Experience Tests Used to Assess Vision', *BMJ Open* 9 (3), (2019): e020905. https://doi.org/10.1136/bmjopen-2017-020905.

Bowers, A. R.; Keeney, K.; Peli, E. 'Randomized Crossover Clinical Trial of Real and Sham Peripheral Prism Glasses for Hemianopia', *JAMA Ophthalmology* 132 (2), (2014): 214–22. https://doi.org/10.1001/jamaophthalmol.2013.5636.

Boyer, D. S.; Schmidt-Erfurth, U.; van Lookeren Campagne, M.; Henry, E. C.; Brittain, C. 'The Pathophysiology of Geographic Atrophy Secondary to Age-Related Macular Degeneration and the Complement Pathway as a Therapeutic Target', *Retina* 37 (5), (2017): 819–35. https://doi.org/10.1097/IAE.0000000000001392.

Brown, F. E.; Sutton, J.; Yuen, H. M.; Green, D.; Van Dorn, S.; Braun, T.; Cree, A. J.; Russell, S. R.; Lotery, A. J. 'A Novel, Wearable, Electronic Visual Aid to Assist Those with Reduced Peripheral Vision', *PLoS One* 14 (10), (2019): e0223755. https://doi.org/10.1371/journal.pone.0223755.

Browning, B. L.; Browning, S. R. 'Statistical Phasing of 150,119 Sequenced Genomes in the UK Biobank', *American Journal of Human Genetics* 110 (1), (2023): 161–65. https://doi.org/10.1016/j.ajhg.2022.11.008.

Brunes, A.; Flanders, W. D.; Augestad, L. B. 'Physical Activity and Symptoms of Anxiety and Depression in Adults with and without Visual Impairments: The HUNT Study', *Mental Health and Physical Activity* 13 (2017): 49–56. https://doi.org/10.1016/j.mhpa.2017.09.001.

Busaeed, S.; Katib, I.; Albeshri, A.; Corchado, J. M.; Yigitcanlar, T.; Mehmood, R. 'LidSonic V2.0: A LiDAR and Deep-Learning-Based Green Assistive Edge Device to Enhance Mobility for the Visually Impaired', *Sensors* 22 (19), (2022): 7435. https://doi.org/10.3390/s22197435.

Cappagli, G.; Cocchi, E.; Gori, M. 'Auditory and Proprioceptive Spatial Impairments in Blind Children and Adults', *Developmental Science* 20 (3), (2017): e12374. https://doi.org/10.1111/desc.12374.

Carmeliet, P. 'VEGF as a Key Mediator of Angiogenesis in Cancer', *Oncology* 69 Suppl. 3, (2005): 4–10. https://doi.org/10.1159/000088478.

'Carmen Papalia: Mobility Device'. 2013. Accessed 14 December 2022. https://www.youtube.com/watch?v=c687G5ZdRxw.

Chai, Y. X.; Gan, A. T. L.; Fenwick, E. K.; Sui, A. Y.; Tan, B. K. J.; Quek, D. Q. Y.; Qian, C. et al. 'Relationship between Vision Impairment and Employment', *British Journal of Ophthalmology* 107 (3), (2023): 361–66. https://doi.org/10.1136/bjophthalmol-2021-319655.

Chakraborty, I. 'To "The Other Senses": A Dialogue between Visual Arts and Visual Disability', *International Research Journal*, Jadavpur University Centre for Disability Studies, IV (2018): 1–8.

Chan, C.-C. 'Couching for Cataract in China', *Survey of Ophthalmology* 55 (4), (2010): 393–98. https://doi.org/10.1016/j.survophthal.2010.02.001.

Chen, B. S.; Yu-Wai-Man, P.; Newman, N. J. 'Developments in the Treatment of Leber Hereditary Optic Neuropathy', *Current Neurology and Neuroscience Reports* 22 (12), (2022): 881–92. https://doi.org/10.1007/s11910-022-01246-y.

Chen, P. P. 'Blindness in Patients with Treated Open-Angle Glaucoma', *Ophthalmology* 110 (4), (2003): 726–33. https://doi.org/10.1016/S0161-6420(02)01974-7.

Cheong, A. M. Y.; Legge, G. E.; Lawrence, M. G.; Cheung, S.-H.; Ruff, M. A. 'Relationship between Slow Visual Processing and Reading Speed in People with Macular Degeneration', *Vision Research* 47 (23), (2007): 2943–55. https://doi.org/10.1016/j.visres.2007.07.010.

Cheung, C. M. G.; Arnold, J. J.; Holz, F. G.; Park, K. H.; Lai, T. Y. Y.; Larsen, M.; Mitchell, P. et al. 'Myopic Choroidal Neovascularization: Review, Guidance, and Consensus Statement on Management', *Ophthalmology* 124 (11), (2017): 1690–1711. https://doi.org/10.1016/j.ophtha.2017.04.028.

Cheung, S.-H.; Fang, F.; He, S.; Legge, G. E. 'Retinotopically Specific Reorganization of Visual Cortex for Tactile Pattern Recognition', *Current Biology* 19 (7), (2009): 596–601. https://doi.org/10.1016/j.cub.2009.02.063.

Chevigny, H.; Braverman, S. *The Adjustment of the Blind*. New Haven: Yale University Press, 1950.

Clayton, L. 'Sculpture for the Blind, by the Blind'. Accessed 31 March 2022. http://www.lenkaclayton.com/work#/sculpture-for-the-blind-by-the-blind.

CNIB Foundation. 'Employment. Know Your Rights – CNIB', 2019. https://www.cnib.ca/en/employment-handbook-ontario?region=on. Accessed on 22 June 2022.

Cohen, P. 'Marriage Rates among People with Disabilities (Save the Data Edition)', Council on Contemporary Families. https://thesocietypages.org/ccf/2014/11/24/marriage-rates-among-people-with-disabilities-save-the-data-edition. Accessed 10 January 2023.

Cohen, P. 'People with Disabilities Are More Likely to Get Divorced', Family Inequality. https://familyinequality.wordpress.com/2013/03/16/disabilities-divorce. Accessed 10 January 2023.

Coletti Moja, M.; Milano, E.; Gasverde, S.; Gianelli, M.; Giordana, M. T. 'Olanzapine Therapy in Hallucinatory Visions Related to Bonnet Syndrome', *Neurological Sciences* 26 (3), (2005): 168–70. https://doi.org/10.1007/s10072-005-0455-0.

Cooney, G. M.; Dwan, K.; Greig, C. A.; Lawlor, D. A.; Rimer, J.; Waugh, F. R.; McMurdo, M.; Mead, G. E. 'Exercise for Depression', *Cochrane Database of Systematic Reviews* 9, (2013). https://doi.org/10.1002/14651858.CD004366.pub6.

Corn, A. L.; Erin, J. N. *Foundations of Low Vision: Clinical and Functional Perspectives*. Louisville: American Printing House for the Blind, 2010.

Crabb, D. P.; Smith, N. D.; Glen, F. C.; Burton, R.; Garway-Heath, D. F. 'How Does Glaucoma Look?: Patient Perception of Visual Field Loss', *Ophthalmology* 120 (6), (2013): 1120–26. https://doi.org/10.1016/j.ophtha.2012.11.043.

Crossland, M. D.; Culham, L. E.; Kabanarou, S. A.; Rubin, G. S. 'Preferred Retinal Locus Development in Patients with Macular Disease', *Ophthalmology* 112 (9), (2005): 1579–85. https://doi.org/10.1016/j.ophtha.2005.03.027.

Crossland, M. D.; Starke, S. D.; Imielski, P.; Wolffsohn, J. S.; Webster, A. R. 'Benefit of an Electronic Head-Mounted Low Vision Aid', *Ophthalmic Physiological Optics* 39 (6), (2019): 422–31. https://doi.org/10.1111/opo.12646.

Crossland, M. D.; Reuben, M.; Bedford, S. L. 'Novel Use of a Franklin Split Lens for Cycling with Hemianopia', *Ophthalmic and Physiological Optics* 42 (1), (2022): 218–23. https://doi.org/10.1111/OPO.12906.

Cumberland, P. M.; Rahi, J. S. 'UK Biobank Eye and Vision Consortium. Visual Function, Social Position, and Health and Life Chances: The UK Biobank Study', *JAMA Ophthalmology* 134 (9), (2016): 959–66. https://doi.org/10.1001/jamaophthalmol.2016.1778.

da Cruz, L.; Fynes, K.; Georgiadis, O.; Kerby, J.; Luo, Y. H.; Ahmado, A.; Vernon, A. et al. 'Phase 1 Clinical Study of an Embryonic Stem Cell-Derived Retinal Pigment Epithelium Patch in Age-Related Macular Degeneration', *Nature Biotechnology* 36 (4), (2018): 328–37. https://doi.org/10.1038/nbt.4114.

Dakin, S.; Carlin, P.; Hemsley, D. 'Weak Suppression of Visual Context in Chronic Schizophrenia', *Current Biology* 15 (20), (2005): R822–24. https://doi.org/10.1016/j.cub.2005.10.015.

Dale, N.; Sakkalou, E.; Osborne, J. 'Early Years, Early Intervention, and Family Support'. In *Children with Vision Impairment: Assessment, Development, and Management*, edited by Dale, N.; Salt, A.; Sargent, J. and Greenaway, R. London: Mac Keith Press, 2021.

Danckert, J.; Striemer, C.; Rossetti, Y. 'Blindsight', *Handbook of Clinical Neurology* 178, (2021): 297–310. https://doi.org/10.1016/B978-0-12-821377-3.00016-7.

Davis, T. R. 'Miners' Nystagmus', *Journal of Hand Surgery* 26 (5), (2001): 399–400. https://doi.org/10.1054/jhsb.2001.0667.

De Fauw, J.; Ledsam, J. R.; Romera-Paredes, B.; Nikolov, S.; Tomasev, N.; Blackwell, S.; Askham, H. et al. 'Clinically Applicable Deep Learning for Diagnosis and Referral in Retinal Disease', *Nature Medicine* 24 (9), (2018): 1342–50. https://doi.org/10.1038/s41591-018-0107-6.

Deemer, A. D.; Bradley, C. K.; Ross, N. C.; Natale, D. M.; Itthipanichpong, R.; Werblin, F. S.; Massof, R. W. 'Low Vision Enhancement with Head-Mounted Video Display Systems: Are We There Yet?', *Optometry and Vision Science* 95 (9), (2018): 694–703. https://doi.org/10.1097/OPX.0000000000001278.

Department of Health. 'Certificate of Vision Impairment: Explanatory Notes for Consultant Ophthalmologists and Hospital Eye Clinic Staff in England, 2017'. https://assets.publishing.

service.gov.uk/government/uploads/system/uploads/attachment_data/file/637590/CVI_guidance.pdf. Accessed 8 March 2022.

DREDF. 'India – The Rights of Persons with Disabilities Act 2016'. https://dredf.org/legal-advocacy/international-disability-rights/international-laws/india-the-rights-of-persons-with-disabilities-act-2016. Accessed 22 June 2022.

Dunn, A. L.; Trivedi, M. H.; Kampert, J. B.; Clark, C. G.; Chambliss, H. O. 'Exercise Treatment for Depression: Efficacy and Dose Response', *American Journal of Preventive Medicine* 28 (1), (2005): 1–8. https://doi.org/10.1016/j.amepre.2004.09.003.

Durr, N. J.; Dave, S. R.; Lage, E.; Marcos, S.; Thorn, F.; Lim, D. 'From Unseen to Seen: Tackling the Global Burden of Uncorrected Refractive Errors', *Annual Review of Biomedical Engineering* 16 (2014): 131–53. https://doi.org/10.1146/annurev-bioeng-071813-105216.

Elementary Education (Blind and Deaf Children) Act 1893 (Circular 347), 21.

'Esme's Umbrella'. Accessed 11 October 2022. https://charlesbonnetsyndrome.uk.

Farahbakhsh, M.; Anderson, E. J.; Maimon-Mor, R. O.; Rider, A.; Greenwood, J. A.; Hirji, N.; Zaman, S. et al. 'A Demonstration of Cone Function Plasticity after Gene Therapy in Achromatopsia', *Brain* 145 (11), (2022): 3803–15. https://doi.org/10.1093/brain/awac226.

Farraher, J. J.; Friedrichsen, T.; Fitzgibbons, R. P. 'Masturbation', In *New Catholic Encyclopedia Supplement 2012–2013: Ethics and Philosophy*, Vol. 3. Farmington Hills: Gale, 2013.

Fenby, E. *Delius as I Knew Him*. London: Icon Books, 1966.

Fernandez-Viadero, C.; Crespo, D.; Verduga, R. 'Necker's Cube a New Tool in Dementia Evaluation', *Neurobiology of Aging* 21, (2000): 30. https://doi.org/10.1016/S0197-4580(00)82811-0.

Ferrey, A.; Moore, L.; Jolly, J. K. '"It Was like Being Hit with a Brick": A Qualitative Study on the Effect of Clinicians' Delivery of a Diagnosis of Eye Disease for Patients in Primary and Secondary Care', *BMJ Open* 12 (7), (2022): e059970. https://doi.org/10.1136/bmjopen-2021-059970.

Ffytche, D. H. 'Visual Hallucinations and the Charles Bonnet Syndrome', *Current Psychiatry Reports* 7 (3), (2005): 168–79. https://doi.org/10.1007/s11920-005-0050-3.

Ffytche, D. H. 'Visual Hallucinatory Syndromes: Past, Present, and Future', *Dialogues in Clinical Neuroscience* 9 (2), (2007): 173–89. https://www.tandfonline.com/doi/full/10.31887/DCNS.2007.9.2/dffytche.

Fieger, A.; Röder, B.; Teder-Sälejärvi, W.; Hillyard, S. A.; Neville, H. J. 'Auditory Spatial Tuning in Late-Onset Blindness in Humans', *Journal of Cognitive Neuroscience* 18 (2), (2006): 149–57. https://doi.org/10.1162/jocn.2006.18.2.149.

Fischer, M. D.; Michalakis, S.; Wilhelm, B.; Zobor, D.; Muehlfriedel, R.; Kohl, S.; Weisschuh, N. et al. 'Safety and Vision Outcomes of Subretinal Gene Therapy Targeting Cone Photoreceptors in Achromatopsia: A Nonrandomized Controlled Trial', *JAMA Ophthalmology* 138 (6), (2020): 643–51. https://doi.org/10.1001/jamaophthalmol.2020.1032.

Fishman, R. S. 'Dark as a Dungeon: The Rise and Fall of Coal Miners' Nystagmus', *Archives of Ophthalmology* 124 (11), (2006): 1637–44. https://doi.org/10.1001/archopht.124.11.1637.

Flessa, S. 'Cataract Surgery in Low-Income Countries: A Good Deal!', *Healthcare* 10 (12), (2022): 2580. https://doi.org/10.3390/healthcare10122580.

Fletcher, D. C.; Schuchard, R. A. 'Preferred Retinal Loci Relationship to Macular Scotomas in a Low-Vision Population', *Ophthalmology* 104 (4), (1997): 632–38. https://doi.org/10.1016/s0161-6420(97)30260-7.

Fletcher, D. C.; Schuchard, R. A.; Renninger, L. W. 'Patient Awareness of Binocular Central Scotoma in Age-Related Macular Degeneration', *Optometry and Vision Science* 89 (9) (2012): 1395–98. https://doi.org/10.1097/OPX.0b013e318264cc77.

Föcker, J.; Best, A.; Hölig, C.; Röder, B. 'The Superiority in Voice Processing of the Blind Arises from Neural Plasticity at Sensory Processing Stages', *Neuropsychologia* 50 (8), (2012): 2056–67. https://doi.org/10.1016/j.neuropsychologia.2012.05.006.

Forsman, A. K.; Nyqvist, F.; Schierenbeck, I.; Gustafson, Y.; Wahlbeck, K. 'Structural and Cognitive Social Capital and Depression among Older Adults in Two Nordic Regions', *Aging & Mental Health* 16 (6), (2012): 771–79. https://doi.org/10.1080/13607863.2012.667784.

Frank, C. R.; Xiang, X.; Stagg, B. C.; Ehrlich, J. R. 'Longitudinal Associations of Self-Reported Vision Impairment with Symptoms of Anxiety and Depression among Older Adults in the United States', *JAMA Ophthalmology* 137 (7), (2019): 793–800. https://doi.org/10.1001/jamaophthalmol.2019.1085.

Frasnelli, J.; Collignon, O.; Voss, P.; Lepore, F. 'Crossmodal Plasticity in Sensory Loss', *Progress in Brain Research* 191 (2011): 233–49. https://doi.org/10.1016/B978-0-444-53752-2.00002-3.

Friberg, T. R.; Braunstein, R. A.; Bressler, N. M. 'Sudden Visual Loss Associated with Sexual Activity', *Archives of Ophthalmology* 113 (6), (1995): 738–42. https://doi.org/10.1001/archopht.1995.01100060064033.

Fu, D. J.; Faes, L.; Wagner, S. K.; Moraes, G.; Chopra, R.; Patel, P. J.; Balaskas, K. et al. 'Predicting Incremental and Future Visual Change in Neovascular Age-Related Macular Degeneration Using Deep Learning', *Ophthalmology Retina* 5 (11), (2021): 1074–84. https://doi.org/10.1016/j.oret.2021.01.009.

García Fernández, M.; Navarro, J. C.; Castaño, C. G. 'Long-Term Evolution of Valsalva Retinopathy: A Case Series', *Journal of Medical Case Reports* 6 (1), (2012): 346. https://doi.org/10.1186/1752-1947-6-346.

Gazzard, G.; Konstantakopoulou, E.; Garway-Heath, D.; Garg, A.; Vickerstaff, V.; Hunter, R.; Ambler, G. et al. 'Selective Laser Trabeculoplasty versus Eye Drops for First-Line Treatment of Ocular Hypertension and Glaucoma (LiGHT): A Multicentre Randomised Controlled Trial', *The Lancet* 393 (10180), (2019): 1505–16. https://doi.org/10.1016/S0140-6736(18)32213-X.

General Medical Council. 'Your Health Matters'. https://www.gmc-uk.org/concerns/information-for-doctors-under-investigation/support-for-doctors/your-health-matters. Accessed 22 June 2022.

Glynn, R. J.; Seddon, J. M.; Krug, J. H.; Sahagian, C. R.; Chiavelli, M. E.; Campion, E. W. 'Falls in Elderly Patients with Glaucoma', *Archives of Ophthalmology* 109 (2), (1991): 205–10. https://doi.org/10.1001/archopht.1991.01080020051041.

Godin, M. L. *There Plant Eyes: A Personal and Cultural History of Blindness*. New York: Pantheon Books, 2021.

Gordon, K. D.; Felfeli, T. 'Family Physician Awareness of Charles Bonnet Syndrome', *Family Practice* 35 (5), (2018): 595–98. https://doi.org/10.1093/fampra/cmy006.

Gori, M.; Sandini, G.; Martinoli, C.; Burr, D. C. 'Impairment of Auditory Spatial Localization in Congenitally Blind Human Subjects', *Brain* 137 (1), (2014): 288–93. https://doi.org/10.1093/brain/awt311.

Gourgey, C. 'Music Therapy in the Treatment of Social Isolation in Visually Impaired Children', *RE:view* 29 (4), (1998): 157.

Granquist, C.; Sun, S.; Montezuma, S.; Tran, T. M.; Gage, R.; Legge, G. E. 'Evaluation and Comparison of Artificial Intelligence Vision Aids: Orcam MyEye 1 and Seeing AI', *Journal of Visual Impairment & Blindness* 115 (4), (2021): 277–85. https://doi.org/10.1177/0145482X211027.

Granquist, C.; Wu, Y. H.; Gage, R.; Crossland, M. D.; Legge, G. E. 'How People with Low Vision Achieve Magnification in Digital Reading', *Optometry and Vision Science* 95 (9), (2018): 711–19. https://doi.org/10.1097/OPX.0000000000001261.

Grant, P.; Spencer, L.; Arnoldussen, A.; Hogle, R.; Nau, A.; Szlyk, J.; Nussdorf, J. et al. 'The Functional Performance of the BrainPort V100 Device in Persons Who Are Profoundly Blind', *Journal of Visual Impairment & Blindness* 110 (2), (2016): 77–88. https://doi.org/10.1177/0145482X1611000202.

Gregory, R. L.; Wallace, J. G. 'Recovery from Early Blindness: A Case Study', *Experimental Psychology Society Monograph; No.2*. Cambridge: Heffer, 1963. https://www.richardgregory.org/papers/recovery_blind/recovery-from-early-blindness.pdf.

Gregory, R. 'The Blind Leading the Sighted', *Nature* 430 (7002), (2004): 836. https://doi.org/10.1038/430836a.

Griessenauer, C. J.; Salam, S.; Hendrix, P.; Patel, D. M.; Tubbs, R. S.; Blount, J. P.; Winkler, P. A. 'Hemispherectomy for Treatment of Refractory Epilepsy in the Pediatric Age Group: A Systematic Review', *Journal of Neurosurgery Pediatrics* 15 (1), (2015): 34–44. https://doi.org/10.3171/2014.10.PEDS14155.

Grzybowski, A.; Claoué, C.; Schwartz, S. G. 'Extracapsular Cataract Extraction in Europe Prior to Jacques Daviel', *Acta Ophthalmologica* 101, (2023): 349–52. https://doi.org/10.1111/aos.15282.

Grzybowski, A.; Shtayer, C.; Schwartz, S. G.; Moisseiev, E. 'The 100 Most-Cited Papers on Age-Related Macular Degeneration: A Bibliographic Perspective', *BMJ Open Ophthalmology* 6 (1), (2021): e000823. https://doi.org/10.1136/bmjophth-2021-000823.

Guimaraes, T. A. C. de; Georgiou, M.; Bainbridge, J. W. B.; Michaelides, M. 'Gene Therapy for Neovascular Age-Related Macular Degeneration: Rationale, Clinical Trials and Future Directions', *British Journal of Ophthalmology* 105 (2), (2021): 151–57. https://doi.org/10.1136/bjophthalmol-2020-316195.

Gunasekeran, D. V.; Zheng, F.; Lim, G. Y. S.; Chong, C. C. Y.; Zhang, S.; Ng, W. Y.; Keel, S. et al. 'Acceptance and Perception of Artificial Intelligence Usability in Eye Care (APPRAISE) for Ophthalmologists: A Multinational Perspective', *Frontiers in Medicine* 9, (2022): 875242. https://doi.org/10.3389/fmed.2022.875242.

Hadjikhani, N.; de Gelder, B. 'Neural Basis of Prosopagnosia: An fMRI Study', *Human Brain Mapping* 16 (3), (2002): 176–82. https://doi.org/10.1002/hbm.10043.

Hallgren, M.; Kandola, A.; Stubbs, B.; Nguyen, T.-T.-D.; Wallin, P.; Andersson, G.; Ekblom-Bak, E. 'Associations of Exercise Frequency and Cardiorespiratory Fitness with Symptoms of Depression and Anxiety – a Cross-Sectional Study of 36,595 Adults', *Mental Health and Physical Activity* 19 (2020): 100351. https://doi.org/10.1016/j.mhpa.2020.100351.

Hamilton, R. H.; Pascual-Leone, A.; Schlaug, G. 'Absolute Pitch in Blind Musicians', *NeuroReport* 15 (5), (2004): 803–6. https://doi.org/10.1097/00001756-200404090-00012.

Harland, S.; Legge, G. E.; Luebker, A. 'Psychophysics of Reading. XVII. Low-Vision Performance with Four Types of Electronically Magnified Text', *Optometry and Vision Science* 75 (3), (1998): 183–90. https://doi.org/10.1097/00006324-199803000-00023.

Harman, N. B. The Education of High Myopes. Proc R Soc Med 1913, 6 (Sect Ophthalmol), 146–163. https://pubmed.ncbi.nlm.nih.gov/19977269.

Harman, N. B. 'The Education of Children with Defective Vision', *Journal of the Royal Society of Medicine* 8, (1915): 107–122.

Hathaway, W. *Education and Health of the Partially Seeing Child*. New York: Columbia University Press, 1943.

Hawkins, K. 'The Blind Sculptor Who Thinks Everyone Should Touch Art', BBC News. https://www.bbc.co.uk/news/blogs-ouch-29837275. Accessed 31 March 2021.

Heimler, B.; Weisz, N.; Collignon, O. 'Revisiting the Adaptive and Maladaptive Effects of Crossmodal Plasticity', *Neuroscience* 283 (2014): 44–63. https://doi.org/10.1016/j.neuroscience.2014.08.003.

Hewett, R.; Brydon, G. 'Careers Education Information and Guidance Support in England: How Well Does CEIAG in England Support Young People with Vision Impairment When Preparing for Life after School?', Thomas Pocklington Trust, 2020. https://www.pocklington-trust.org.uk/wp-content/uploads/2020/10/CEIAG_Research_Report_-_Overview_-_Final.docx.

Holbrook, M. C.; Zebehazy, K. T. 'Reading Approaches for Braille Readers'. In *Children with Vision Impairment: Assessment, Development and Management*, edited by Naomi Dale, Alison Salt, Jenefer Sargent and Rebecca Greenaway. London: Mac Keith Press, 2022.

Holmström, G. 'Retinopathy of Prematurity', *British Medical Journal* 307 (6906), (1993): 694–95. https://doi.org/10.1136/bmj.307.6906.694.

House of Commons. Board of Education. 'Annual Report for 1918 of the Chief Medical Officer of the Board of Education'. London, 1919.

'How This Blind Girl …', 2022. BBC. https://www.bbc.co.uk/programmes/m001fknv#credits. Accessed 10 January 2023.

Howe, L. 'The Relation of Hereditary Eye Defects to Genetics and Eugenics', *JAMA* 70 (26), (1918): 1994–99. https://doi.org/10.1001/jama.1918.02600260006004.

Hull, J. M. *Touching the Rock: An Experience of Blindness*. London: SPCK, 1990.

International Blind Sports Federation. 'IBSA Classification Manual for Classifiers'. https://ibsasport.org/wp-content/uploads/2020/07/IBSA-Classification-Manual-classifiers.pdf. Accessed 22 June 2022.

Isawumi, M. A.; Kolawole, O. U.; Hassan, M. B. 'Couching Techniques for Cataract Treatment in Osogbo, South West Nigeria', *Ghana Medical Journal* 47 (2), (2013): 64–69. https://www.ncbi.nlm.nih.gov/pmc/articles/PMC3743109.

Ivy, S. E.; Ledford, J. R. 'A Systematic Review of Behavioral Interventions to Reduce Restricted or Repetitive Behavior of Individuals with Visual Impairment', *Journal of Behavioral Education* 31 (1), (2022): 94–122. https://doi.org/10.1007/s10864-020-09418-x.

Jackson, M. L.; Bassett, K.; Nirmalan, P. K. 'Charles Bonnet Hallucinations: Natural History and Risk Factors', *International Congress Series* 1282, (2005): 592–95. https://doi.org/10.1016/j.ics.2005.05.186.

Jefsen, O. H.; Petersen, L. V.; Bek, T.; Østergaard, S. D. 'Is Early Blindness Protective of Psychosis or Are We Turning a Blind Eye to the Lack of Statistical Power?', *Schizophrenia Bulletin* 46 (6), (2020): 1335–36. https://doi.org/10.1093/schbul/sbaa048.

Jin, Z.-B.; Gao, M.-L.; Deng, W.-L.; Wu, K.-C.; Sugita, S.; Mandai, M.; Takahashi, M. 'Stemming Retinal Regeneration with Pluripotent Stem Cells', *Progress in Retinal and Eye Research* 69, (2019): 38–56. https://doi.org/10.1016/j.preteyeres.2018.11.003.

Johnson, D. H. 'Progress in Glaucoma: Early Detection, New Treatments, Less Blindness', *Ophthalmology* 110 (4), (2003): 634–35. https://doi.org/10.1016/S0161-6420(03)00411-1.

Jonas, J. B.; Cheung, C. M. G.; Panda-Jonas, S. 'Updates on the Epidemiology of Age-Related Macular Degeneration', *Asia-Pacific Journal of Ophthalmology* 6 (6), (2017): 493–97. https://doi.org/10.22608/APO.2017251.

Jones, G. 'Echolocation', *Current Biology* 15 (13), (2005): R484–88. https://doi.org/10.1016/j.cub.2005.06.051.

Jones, L.; Moosajee, M. 'Visual Hallucinations and Sight Loss in Children and Young Adults: A Retrospective Case Series of Charles Bonnet Syndrome', *British Journal of Ophthalmology* 105 (11), (2021): 1604–9. https://doi.org/10.1136/bjophthalmol-2020-317237.

Jones, L.; Murray, M.; Gomes, R. S. M. 'Moving Towards Inclusivity: A Call for Increased Speed and Intensity in Making Fitness Facilities Accessible for People with Visual Impairments', *Journal of Visual Impairment & Blindness* 116 (5), (2022): 752–55. https://doi.org/10.1177/0145482X221133938.

Jones, T. 'Estimating the Speed of Vehicles Using an Electronic Travel-Aid Interface', *British Journal of Visual Impairment* 24 (1), (2006): 12–18. https://doi.org/10.1177/02646196 06060029.

Kamourieh, S.; Sokolska, M.; Akram, H.; Patel, J.; Jäger, H. R.; Arshad, Q.; Matharu, M.; Kaski, D. 'Miners' Nystagmus Following Visual Deprivation: A Case Report', *Annals of Internal Medicine* 174 (7), (2021): 1021–22. https://doi.org/10.7326/L20-1261.

Kanazawa, S.; Tsunoda, T.; Onuma, E.; Majima, T.; Kagiyama, M.; Kikuchi, K. 'VEGF, Basic-FGF, and TGF-Beta in Crohn's Disease and Ulcerative Colitis: A Novel Mechanism of Chronic Intestinal Inflammation', *American Journal of Gastroenterology* 96 (3), (2001): 822–28. https://pubmed.ncbi.nlm.nih.gov/11280558.

Kapperman, G. 'On Being Blind'. In *The Routledge Handbook of Visual Impairment,* edited by J. Ravenscroft. London: Routledge, 2019.

Kapperman, G.; Kelly, S. M. 'Human Mate Selection Theory: Specific Considerations for Persons with Visual Impairments'. In *The Routledge Handbook of Visual Impairment*, edited by J. Ravenscroft. London: Routledge, 2019.

Kapperman, G.; Kelly, S. M.; Kilmer, K.; Smith, T. J. 'An Assessment of the Tinder Mobile Dating Application for Individuals Who Are Visually Impaired', *Journal of Visual Impairment and Blindness* 111 (4), (2017): 369–74. https://doi.org/10.1177/0145482X1711100406.

Kef, S.; Bos, H. 'Is Love Blind? Sexual Behavior and Psychological Adjustment of Adolescents with Blindness', *Sexuality and Disability* 24 (2), (2006): 89–100. https://doi.org/10.1007/s11195-006-9007-7.

Keller, B.; Draelos, M.; Zhou, K.; Qian, R.; Kuo, A.; Konidaris, G.; Hauser, K. 'Optical Coherence Tomography-Guided Robotic Ophthalmic Microsurgery via Reinforcement Learning from Demonstration', *IEEE Transactions on Robotics* 36 (4), (2020): 1207–18. https://doi.org/10.1109/TRO.2020.2980158.

Kellner, U.; Bedar, M. S.; Weinitz, S.; Farmand, G.; Sürül, E. N.; Weide, S. M.; Schick, T. 'Treatment Contentment and Preference of Patients Undergoing Intravitreal Anti-VEGF Therapy', *Graefe's Archive for Clinical and Experimental Ophthalmology* 259 (12), (2021): 3649–54. https://doi.org/10.1007/s00417-021-05324-8.

Kelman, C. D. 'Phaco-Emulsification and Aspiration. A New Technique of Cataract Removal. A Preliminary Report', *American Journal of Ophthalmology* 64 (1), (1967): 23–35. doi: 10.1016/j.ajo.2018.04.014.

Kendrick, D. 'Review of "The Blind Doctor: The Jacob Bolotin Story" by Rosalind Perlman', *Braille Monitor* 51 (1), (2008). https://nfb.org/images/nfb/publications/bm/bm08/bm0801/bm0801.htm. Accessed 13 July 2022.

Kenneally, C. 'The Deepest Cut', *The New Yorker*, 25 June 2006. https://www.newyorker.com/magazine/2006/07/03/the-deepest-cut. Accessed 4 October 2022.

Kerr, J. *School Vision and the Myopic Scholar*. London: George Allen and Unwin, 1925.

Keuss, S. E.; Bowen, J.; Schott, J. M. 'Looking beyond the Eyes: Visual Impairment in Posterior Cortical Atrophy', *The Lancet* 394 (10203), (2019): 1055. https://doi.org/10.1016/S0140-6736(19)31818-5.

Khairallah, M.; Kahloun, R.; Bourne, R.; Limburg, H.; Flaxman, S. R.; Jonas, J. B.; Keeffe, J.; Leasher, J.; Naidoo, K.; Pesudovs, K. et al. 'Number of People Blind or Visually Impaired by Cataract Worldwide and in World Regions, 1990 to 2010', *Investigative Ophthalmology & Visual Science* 56 (11), (2015): 6762–69. https://doi.org/10.1167/iovs.15-17201.

Kilcrease, A. '10 Questions with … Chris Downey', *Interior Design*, 6 June 2016. Accessed 19 April 2022. https://interiordesign.net/designwire/10-questions-with-chris-downey.

Kim, L. N.; Cordato, D.; McDougall, A.; Fraser, C. 'Pilot Study: The Queen Square Screening Test for Visual Deficits in Dementia', *Neuro-Ophthalmology* 45 (6), (2021): 380–85. https://doi.org/10.1080/01658107.2021.1947324.

King, N. M.; Perrin, J. 'Ethical Issues in Stem Cell Research and Therapy', *Stem Cell Research and Therapy* 5 (4), (2014): 85. https://doi.org/10.1186/scrt474.

Kirkman, M. A.; Korsten, A.; Leonhardt, M.; Dimitriadis, K.; De Coo, I. F.; Klopstock, T.; Griffiths, P. G.; Hudson, G.; Chinnery, P. F.; Yu-Wai-Man, P. 'Quality of Life in Patients with Leber Hereditary Optic Neuropathy', *Investigative Ophthalmology and Visual Science* 50 (7), (2009): 3112–15. https://doi.org/10.1167/iovs.08-3166.

Kleege, G. *More than Meets the Eye: What Blindness Brings to Art*. Oxford: Oxford University Press, 2018.

Kleege, G. *Sight Unseen*. New Haven: Yale University Press, 1999.

Kornmeier, J.; Bach, M. 'The Necker Cube – an Ambiguous Figure Disambiguated in Early Visual Processing', *Vision Research* 45 (8), (2005): 955–60. https://doi.org/10.1016/j.visres.2004.10.006.

Kroenke, K.; Spitzer, R. L.; Williams, J. B. W. 'The Patient Health Questionnaire-2: Validity of a Two-Item Depression Screener', *Medical Care* 41 (11), (2003): 1284–92. https://doi.org/10.1097/01.MLR.0000093487.78664.3C.

Kupers, R.; Beaulieu-Lefebvre, M.; Schneider, F. C.; Kassuba, T.; Paulson, O. B.; Siebner, H. R.; Ptito, M. 'Neural Correlates of Olfactory Processing in Congenital Blindness', *Neuropsychologia* 49 (7), (2011): 2037–44. https://doi.org/10.1016/j.neuropsychologia.2011.03.033.

Kurson, R. *Crashing Through: A True Story of Risk, Adventure and the Man Who Dared to See*. New York: Random House, 2007.

Kuusisto, S. *Eavesdropping: A Memoir of Blindness and Listening*. London: W.W. Norton, 2006.

Kuusisto, S. *Planet of the Blind*. London: Faber and Faber, 1998.

KV, V.; Vijayalakshmi, P. 'Understanding Definitions of Visual Impairment and Functional Vision', *Community Eye Health* 33 (110), (2020): S16–17. https://www.ncbi.nlm.nih.gov/pmc/articles/PMC8115704/.

Lam, B. L.; Christ, S. L.; Lee, D. J.; Zheng, D. D.; Arheart, K. L. 'Reported Visual Impairment and Risk of Suicide: The 1986–1996 National Health Interview Surveys', *Archives of Ophthalmology* 126 (7), (2008): 975–80. https://doi.org/10.1001/archopht.126.7.975.

Lang, U. E.; Stogowski, D.; Schulze, D.; Domula, M.; Schmidt, E.; Gallinat, J.; Tugtekin, S. M.; Felber, W. 'Charles Bonnet Syndrome: Successful Treatment of Visual Hallucinations Due to Vision Loss with Selective Serotonin Reuptake Inhibitors', *Journal of Psychopharmacology* 21 (5), (2007): 553–56. https://doi.org/10.1177/0269881106075.

Laqueur, T. W. *Solitary Sex: A Cultural History of Masturbation*. New York: Zone Books, 2003.

'Latanoprost Ophthalmic Prices, Coupons and Patient Assistance Programs', Drugs.com. Accessed 31 January 2023. https://www.drugs.com/price-guide/latanoprost-ophthalmic.

Laukkonen, R. E.; Tangen, J. M. 'Can Observing a Necker Cube Make You More Insightful?', *Consciousness and Cognition* 48 (2017): 198–211. https://doi.org/10.1016/j.concog.2016.11.011.

Leat, S. J. 'To Prescribe or Not To Prescribe? Guidelines for Spectacle Prescribing in Infants and Children', *Clinical and Experimental Optometry* 94 (6), (2011): 514–27. https://doi.org/10.1111/j.1444-0938.2011.00600.x.

Lee, O. E.-K.; Park, D.; Park, J. 'Association of Vision Impairment with Suicide Ideation, Plans, and Attempts among Adults in the United States', *Journal of Clinical Psychology* 78 (11), (2022): 2197–2213. https://doi.org/10.1002/jclp.23437.

Leffler, C. T.; Klebanov, A.; Samara, W. A.; Grzybowski, A. 'The History of Cataract Surgery: From Couching to Phacoemulsification', *Annals of Translational Medicine* 8 (22), (2020): 1551. https://doi.org/10.21037/atm-2019-rcs-04.

Leffler, C. T.; Schwartz, S. G.; Peterson, E.; Couser, N. L.; Salman, A.-R. 'The First Cataract Surgeons in the British Isles', *American Journal of Ophthalmology* 230, (2021): 75–122. https://doi.org/10.1016/j.ajo.2021.03.009.

Legge, G. E. *Psychophysics of Reading in Normal and Low Vision*. Mahwah: Lawrence Erlbaum Associates, 2007.

Legge, G. E.; Ahn, S. J.; Klitz, T. S.; Luebker, A. 'Psychophysics of Reading – XVI. The Visual Span in Normal and Low Vision', *Vision Research* 37 (14), (1997): 1999–2010. https://doi.org/10.1016/S0042-6989(97)00017-5.

Legge, G. E.; Bigelow, C. A. 'Does Print Size Matter for Reading? A Review of Findings from Vision Science and Typography', *Journal of Vision* 11 (5), (2011): 8. https://doi.org/10.1167/11.5.8.

Legge, G. E.; Granquist, C.; Lubet, A.; Gage, R.; Xiong, Y.-Z. 'Preserved Tactile Acuity in Older Pianists', *Attention, Perception, & Psychophysics* 81 (8), (2019): 2619–25. https://doi.org/10.3758/s13414-019-01844-y.

Legge, G. E.; Madison, C.; Vaughn, B. N.; Cheong, A. M. Y.; Miller, J. C. 'Retention of High Tactile Acuity Throughout the Lifespan in Blindness', *Perception & Psychophysics* 70 (8), (2008): 1471–88. https://doi.org/10.3758/PP.70.8.1471.

Leivada, E.; Boeckx, C. 'Schizophrenia and Cortical Blindness: Protective Effects and Implications for Language', *Frontiers in Human Neuroscience* 8 (2014): 940. https://doi.org/10.3389/fnhum.2014.00940.

Leland, A. 'Feeling Seen', *New York Times Magazine*, 4 July 2021 (2021): 34–45. https://www.nytimes.com/2021/07/01/magazine/in-the-dark-blindness.html?searchResultPosition=1.

Lewald, J. 'Exceptional Ability of Blind Humans to Hear Sound Motion: Implications for the Emergence of Auditory Space', *Neuropsychologia* 51 (1), (2013): 181–86. https://doi.org/10.1016/j.neuropsychologia.2012.11.017.

Li, F.; Chen, H.; Liu, Z.; Zhang, X.; Wu, Z. 'Fully Automated Detection of Retinal Disorders by Image-Based Deep Learning', *Graefe's Archive for Clinical and Experimental Ophthalmology* 257 (3), (2019): 495–505. https://doi.org/10.1007/s00417-018-04224-8.

Liao, D. S.; Grossi, F. V.; El Mehdi, D.; Gerber, M. R.; Brown, D. M.; Heier, J. S.; Wykoff, C. C. et al. 'Complement C3 Inhibitor Pegcetacoplan for Geographic Atrophy Secondary to Age-Related Macular Degeneration: A Randomized Phase 2 Trial', *Ophthalmology* 127 (2), (2020): 186–95. https://doi.org/10.1016/j.ophtha.2019.07.011.

Liotti, M.; Ryder, K.; Woldorff, M. G. 'Auditory Attention in the Congenitally Blind: Where, When and What Gets Reorganized?', *NeuroReport* 9 (6), (1998): 1007–12. https://doi.org/10.1097/00001756-199804200-00010.

Living Paintings. 'Our Books'. https://livingpaintings.org/books. Accessed 19 April 2022.

Living Paintings. Trustees' Report and Financial Statements 2019–20. https://livingpaintings.org/wp-content/uploads/2021/06/Living-Paintings-Directors-Report-and-Accounts-1st-June-2019-31st-May-2020.pdf. Accessed 19 April 2022.

Llewellyn, T. L. 'A Lecture on Miners' Nystagmus', *British Medical Journal* 1 (2739), (1913): 1359–61. https://doi.org/10.1136/bmj.1.2739.1359.

Loued-Khenissi, L.; Preuschoff, K. 'A Bird's Eye View from Below: Activity in the Temporo-Parietal Junction Predicts from-above Necker Cube Percepts', *Neuropsychologia* 149, (2020): 107654. https://doi.org/10.1016/j.neuropsychologia.2020.107654.

Lusseyran, J. *And There Was Light* (Translated by Elizabeth R. Cameron). London: Heinemann, 1963.

Lynskey, D. *33 Revolutions per Minute: A History of Protest Songs*. London: Faber and Faber, 2012.

Mackay, G. J.; Neill, J. T. 'The Effect of "Green Exercise" on State Anxiety and the Role of Exercise Duration, Intensity, and Greenness: A Quasi-Experimental Study', *Psychology of Sport and Exercise* 11 (3), (2010): 238–45. https://doi.org/10.1016/j.psychsport.2010.01.002.

MacLaren, R. E.; Groppe, M.; Barnard, A. R.; Cottriall, C. L.; Tolmachova, T.; Seymour, L.; Clark, K. R. et al. 'Retinal Gene Therapy in Patients with Choroideremia: Initial Findings from a Phase 1/2 Clinical Trial', *The Lancet* 383 (9923), (2014): 1129–37. https://doi.org/10.1016/S0140-6736(13)62117-0.

Macular Society. 'Treatments'. Accessed 7 February 2023. https://www.macularsociety.org/diagnosis-treatment/treatments.

Maguire, A. M.; Simonelli, F.; Pierce, E. A.; Pugh, E. N.; Mingozzi, F.; Bennicelli, J.; Banfi, S. et al. 'Safety and Efficacy of Gene Transfer for Leber's Congenital Amaurosis', *New England Journal of Medicine* 358 (21), (2008): 2240–48. https://doi.org/10.1056/NEJMoa0802315.

Mansfield, J. S.; Legge, G. E.; Bane, M. C. 'Psychophysics of Reading. XV: Font Effects in Normal and Low Vision', *Investigative Ophthalmology & Visual Science* 37 (8), (1996): 1492–1501. https://pubmed.ncbi.nlm.nih.gov/8675391.

Marks, D. 'Models of Disability', *Disability and Rehabilitation* 19 (3), (1997): 85–91. https://doi.org/10.3109/09638289709166831.

Martinsen, E. W. 'Physical Activity in the Prevention and Treatment of Anxiety and Depression', *Nordic Journal of Psychiatry* 62 (S47), (2008): 25–29. https://doi.org/10.1080/08039480802315640.

Massof, R. W.; Rickman, D. L. 'Obstacles Encountered in the Development of the Low Vision Enhancement System', *Optometry and Vision Science* 69 (1), (1992): 32–41. https://doi.org/10.1097/00006324-199201000-00005.

McCarty, C. A.; Burgess, M.; Keeffe, J. E. 'Unemployment and Under-Employment in Adults with Vision Impairment: The RVIB Employment Survey', *Australian and New Zealand Journal of Ophthalmology* 27 (3–4), (1999): 190–93. https://doi.org/10.1046/j.1440-1606.1999.00194.x.

McKenzie, L. E.; Polur, R. N.; Wesley, C.; Allen, J. D.; McKeown, R. E.; Zhang, J. 'Social Contacts and Depression in Middle and Advanced Adulthood: Findings from a US National Survey, 2005–2008', *International Journal of Social Psychiatry* 59 (7), (2013): 627–35. https://doi.org/10.1177/0020764012463302.

'Meet Nobuyuki Tsujii, the Blind Concert Pianist Who Learns by Ear'. https://www.youtube.com/watch?v=kNljZvnByfQ. Accessed 11 May 2022.

Mellor, C. M. *Louis Braille: A Touch of Genius*. Boston: National Braille Press, 2006.

'Mind Changers. Case Study: SB – The Man Who Was Disappointed with What He Saw', 2010. https://www.bbc.co.uk/programmes/b00tgd1g.

Minton, J. *Occupational Eye Diseases and Injuries*. London: William Heinemann Medical Books, 1949.

Mounsey, C. 'Learning from Blindness', *PMLA* 130 (5), (2015): 1506–9. https://doi.org/10.1632/pmla.2015.130.5.1506.

Murray, G. 'Blind Mystic Baba Vanga Who Predicted 9/11 Said Putin Will Be "Lord of the World"', *Daily Mirror*, 26 March 2022. https://www.mirror.co.uk/news/world-news/blind-mystic-baba-vanga-who-26562978. Accessed 28 September 2022.

National Institute for Health and Care Excellence. 'Depression in Adults: Treatment and Management', 2022. https://www.nice.org.uk/guidance/ng222/resources/depression-in-adults-treatment-and-management-pdf-66143832307909. Accessed 30 November 2022.

National Institute for Health and Care Excellence. 'Glaucoma: Diagnosis and Management', 2017. https://www.nice.org.uk/guidance/ng81. Accessed 31 January 2023.

National Institute for Health and Care Excellence. 'Voretigene Neparvovec for Treating Inherited Retinal Dystrophies Caused by RPE65 Gene Mutations', 2019. https://www.nice.org.uk/guidance/hst11/resources/voretigene-neparvovec-for-treating-inherited-retinal-dystrophies-caused-by-rpe65-gene-mutations-pdf-50216253809605. Accessed 28 February 2023.

Neat, L.; Peng, R.; Qin, S.; Manduchi, R. 'Scene Text Access: A Comparison of Mobile OCR Modalities for Blind Users', *IUI International Conference on Intelligent User Interfaces* (2019): 197–207. https://doi.org/10.1145/3301275.3302271.

Nelson, W. L.; Fraunfelder, F. T.; Sills, J. M.; Arrowsmith, J. B.; Kuritsky, J. N. 'Adverse Respiratory and Cardiovascular Events Attributed to Timolol Ophthalmic Solution, 1978–85', *American Journal of Ophthalmology* 102 (5), (1986): 606–11. https://doi.org/10.1016/0002-9394(86)90532-5.

Newman-Casey, P. A.; Robin, A. L.; Blachley, T.; Farris, K.; Heisler, M.; Resnicow, K.; Lee, P. P. 'The Most Common Barriers to Glaucoma Medication Adherence: A Cross-Sectional Survey', *Ophthalmology* 122 (7), (2015): 1308–16. https://doi.org/10.1016/j.ophtha.2015.03.026.

Nguyen, X.-T.-A.; Koopman, J.; van Genderen, M. M.; Stam, H. L. M.; Boon, C. J. F. 'Artificial Vision: The Effectiveness of the OrCam in Patients with Advanced Inherited Retinal Dystrophies', *Acta Ophthalmologica* 100 (4), (2022): e986–93. https://doi.org/10.1111/aos.15001.

NHS England. 'NHS Genomic Medicine Service'. Accessed 31 January 2023. https://www.england.nhs.uk/genomics/nhs-genomic-med-service.

Nishimura, H.; Hashikawa, K.; Doi, K.; Iwaki, T.; Watanabe, Y.; Kusuoka, H.; Nishimura, T.; Kubo, T. 'Sign Language "Heard" in the Auditory Cortex', *Nature* 397 (1999): 116. https://doi.org/10.1038/16376.

Nkrumah, B. 'The Hunted: UDHR and Africans with Albinism', *International Migration* 57 (1), (2019): 192–212. https://doi.org/10.1111/imig.12521.

Nollett, C. L.; Bray, N.; Bunce, C.; Casten, R. J.; Edwards, R. T.; Hegel, M. T.; Janikoun, S. et al. 'Depression in Visual Impairment Trial (DEPVIT): A Randomized Clinical Trial of Depression Treatments in People with Low Vision', *Investigative Ophthalmology & Visual Science* 57 (10), (2016): 4247–54. https://doi.org/10.1167/iovs.16-19345.

Nommiste, B.; Fynes, K.; Tovell, V. E.; Ramsden, C.; da Cruz, L.; Coffey, P. 'Stem Cell-Derived Retinal Pigment Epithelium Transplantation for Treatment of Retinal Disease', *Progress in Brain Research* 231, (2017): 225–44. https://doi.org/10.1016/bs.pbr.2017.03.003.

Nordstrom, B. L.; Friedman, D. S.; Mozaffari, E.; Quigley, H. A.; Walker, A. M. 'Persistence and Adherence with Topical Glaucoma Therapy', *American Journal of Ophthalmology* 140 (4), (2005): 598–606. https://doi.org/10.1016/j.ajo.2005.04.051.

Norman, L. J.; Dodsworth, C.; Foresteire, D.; Thaler, L. 'Human Click-Based Echolocation: Effects of Blindness and Age, and Real-Life Implications in a 10-Week Training Program', *PLoS ONE* 16 (6), (2021): e0252330. https://doi.org/10.1371/journal.pone.0252330.

Norridge, C. F. E.; Gruska-Goh, M. H.; McKibbin, M.; Henry, P.; Donachie, J. 'National Ophthalmology Database Audit: The First Report of Age-Related Macular Degeneration Audit (AMD) for Patients Starting Treatment for Neovascular AMD in the 2020 NHS Year: 01 April 2020 to 31 March 2021', Royal College of Ophthalmologists, 2023. https://nodaudit.org.uk/public/publications. Accessed 21 February 2023.

Notredame, C.-E.; Pins, D.; Deneve, S.; Jardri, R. 'What Visual Illusions Teach Us about Schizophrenia', *Frontiers in Integrative Neuroscience* 8, (2014): 63. https://doi.org/10.3389/fnint.2014.00063.

O'Hare, F.; Edwards, T. L.; Hu, M. L.; Hickey, D. G.; Zhang, A. C.; Wang, J.-H.; Liu, Z.; Ayton, L. N. 'An Optometrist's Guide to the Top Candidate Inherited Retinal Diseases for Gene Therapy', *Clinical and Experimental Optometry* 104 (4), (2021): 431–43. https://doi.org/10.1080/08164622.2021.1878851.

O'Sullivan, S. *It's All in Your Head: True Stories of Imaginary Illness*. London: Random House, 2016.

Odame, L.; Opoku, M. P.; Nketsia, W.; Swanzy, P.; Alzyoudi, M.; Nsowah, F. A. 'From University-to-Work: An In-Depth Exploration into the Transition Journey of Graduates with Sensory Disabilities in Ghana', *Disability & Society* 36 (9), (2021): 1399–422. https://doi.org/10.1080/09687599.2020.1804328.

Office for National Statistics. 'Births in England and Wales: Summary Tables', 2022. Accessed 10 January 2023. https://www.ons.gov.uk/peoplepopulationandcommunity/birthsdeathsandmarriages/livebirths/datasets/birthsummarytables.

Olthoff, C. M. G.; Hoevenaars, J. G. M. M.; van den Borne, B. W.; Webers, C. A. B.; Schouten, J. S. A. G. 'Prevalence and Determinants of Non-Adherence to Topical Hypotensive Treatment in Dutch Glaucoma Patients', *Graefe's Archive for Clinical and Expermintal Ophthalmology* 247 (2), (2009): 235–43. https://doi.org/10.1007/s00417-008-0944-y.

'Onania or, the Heinous Sin of Self-Pollution, and All Its Frightful Consequences, (in Both Sexes) Consider'd'. London, 1730.

'Onanism: Or, a Treatise upon the Disorders Produced by Masturbation'. London, 1781.

Oshima, K.; Arai, T.; Ichihara, S.; Nakano, Y. 'Tactile Sensitivity and Braille Reading in People with Early Blindness and Late Blindness', *Journal of Visual Impairment & Blindness* 108 (2), (2014): 122–32. https://doi.org/10.1177/0145482X1410800204.

Owen, C. G.; Jarrar, Z.; Wormald, R.; Cook, D. G.; Fletcher, A. E.; Rudnicka, A. R. 'The Estimated Prevalence and Incidence of Late Stage Age Related Macular Degeneration in the UK', *British Journal of Ophthalmology* 96 (5), (2012): 752–56. https://doi.org/10.1136/bjophthalmol-2011-301109.

Pałgan, K.; Bartuzi, Z. 'Angiogenesis in Bronchial Asthma', *International Journal of Immunopathology and Pharmacology* 28 (3), (2015): 415–20. https://doi.org/10.1177/0394632015580907.

Paulig, M.; Mentrup, H. 'Charles Bonnet's Syndrome: Complete Remission of Complex Visual Hallucinations Treated by Gabapentin', *Journal of Neurology, Neurosurgery & Psychiatry* 70 (6), (2001): 813–14. https://doi.org/10.1136/jnnp.70.6.813.

Peat, L.; Higgins, N. 'Safe Access to Road Crossings and the Issue of Quiet Vehicles in Relation to Pedestrians with a Vision Impairment: A Literature Review', *British Journal of Visual Impairment* (2022): 26461962211112. https://doi.org/10.1177/02646196221111282.

Pieniak, M.; Lachowicz-Tabaczek, K.; Karwowski, M.; Oleszkiewicz, A. 'Sensory Compensation Beliefs among Blind and Sighted Individuals', *Scandinavian Journal of Psychology* 63 (1), (2022): 72–82. https://doi.org/10.1111/sjop.12781.

Pinquart, M.; Pfeiffer, J. P. 'What Is Essential Is Invisible to the Eye: Intimate Relationships of Adolescents with Visual Impairment', *Sexuality and Disability* 30 (2), (2012): 139–47. https://doi.org/10.1007/s11195-011-9248-y.

Polidoro, R. B.; Hagan, R. S.; de Santis Santiago, R.; Schmidt, N. W. 'Overview: Systemic Inflammatory Response Derived from Lung Injury Caused by SARS-CoV-2 Infection Explains Severe Outcomes in COVID-19', *Frontiers in Immunology* 11, (2020): 1626. https://doi.org/10.3389/fimmu.2020.01626.

Pollak, T. A.; Corlett, P. R. 'Blindness, Psychosis, and the Visual Construction of the World', *Schizophrenia Bulletin* 46 (6), (2020): 1418–25. https://doi.org/10.1093/schbul/sbz098.

Porter, R. *London: A Social History*. London: Penguin, 2000.

Pritchard, D. G. *Education and the Handicapped, 1760–1960*. London: Routledge and Kegan Paul, 1963.

Pundlik, S.; Baliutaviciute, V.; Moharrer, M.; Bowers, A. R.; Luo, G. 'Home-Use Evaluation of a Wearable Collision Warning Device for Individuals with Severe Vision Impairments: A Randomized Clinical Trial', *JAMA Ophthalmology* 139 (9), (2021): 998–1005. https://doi.org/10.1001/jamaophthalmol.2021.2624.

Puomila, A.; Hämäläinen, P.; Kivioja, S.; Savontaus, M.-L.; Koivumäki, S.; Huoponen, K.; Nikoskelainen, E. 'Epidemiology and Penetrance of Leber Hereditary Optic Neuropathy in Finland', *European Journal of Human Genetics* 15 (10), (2007): 1079–89. https://doi.org/10.1038/sj.ejhg.5201828.

Ragert, P.; Schmidt, A.; Altenmüller, E.; Dinse, H. R. 'Superior Tactile Performance and Learning in Professional Pianists: Evidence for Meta-Plasticity in Musicians', *European Journal of Neuroscience* 19 (2), (2004): 473–78. https://doi.org/10.1111/j.0953-816x.2003.03142.x.

Rahi, J.; Logan, S.; Timms, C.; Russell-Eggitt, I.; Taylor, D. 'Risk, Causes, and Outcomes of Visual Impairment after Loss of Vision in the Non-Amblyopic Eye: A Population-Based Study', *The Lancet*, 360 (9333), (2002): 597–602. https://doi.org/10.1016/s0140-6736(02)09782-9.

Rahman, F.; Zekite, A.; Bunce, C.; Jayaram, H.; Flanagan, D. 'Recent Trends in Vision Impairment Certifications in England and Wales', *Eye* 34 (7), (2020): 1271–78. https://doi.org/10.1038/s41433-020-0864-6.

Rahman, M. S.; Yoshida, N.; Hanafusa, M.; Matsuo, A.; Zhu, S.; Stub, Y.; Takahashi, C. et al. 'Screening and Quantification of Undeclared $PGF_{2\alpha}$ Analogs in Eyelash-Enhancing Cosmetic Serums Using LC-MS/MS', *Journal of Pharmaceutical and Biomedical Analysis* 219, (2022): 114940. https://doi.org/10.1016/j.jpba.2022.114940.

Ravin, J. G.; Stern, A. M. 'Lucien Howe, Hereditary Blindness, and the Eugenics Movement', *JAMA Ophthalmology* 128 (7), (2010): 924–30. https://doi.org/10.1001/archophthalmol.2010.137.

Renier, L.; Cuevas, I.; Grandin, C. B.; Dricot, L.; Plaza, P.; Lerens, E.; Rombaux, P.; De Volder, A. G. 'Right Occipital Cortex Activation Correlates with Superior Odor Processing Performance in the Early Blind', *PLoS One* 8 (8), (2013): e71907. https://doi.org/10.1371/journal.pone.0071907.

Resnikoff, S.; Lansingh, V. C.; Washburn, L.; Felch, W.; Gauthier, T.-M.; Taylor, H. R.; Eckert, K.; Parke, D.; Wiedemann, P. 'Estimated Number of Ophthalmologists Worldwide (International Council of Ophthalmology Update): Will We Meet the Needs?', *British Journal of Ophthalmology* 104 (4), (2020): 588. http://dx.doi.org/10.1136/bjophthalmol-2019-314336.

Ribowsky, M. *Signed, Sealed, and Delivered: The Soulful Journey of Stevie Wonder*. Hoboken: John Wiley & Sons, 2010.

Roberts, J. *A Sense of the World: How a Blind Man Became History's Greatest Traveler*. London: Simon and Schuster, 2006.

Rombaux, P.; Huart, C.; De Volder, A. G.; Cuevas, I.; Renier, L.; Duprez, T.; Grandin, C. 'Increased Olfactory Bulb Volume and Olfactory Function in Early Blind Subjects', *NeuroReport* 21 (17), (2010): 1069–73. https://doi.org/10.1097/WNR.0b013e32833fcb8a.

Roos, S. 'The Kübler-Ross Model: An Esteemed Relic', *Gestalt Review* 16 (3), (2012): 312–15. https://doi.org/10.5325/gestaltreview.16.3.0312.

Rose, K. A.; Morgan, I. G.; Ip, J.; Kifley, A.; Huynh, S.; Smith, W.; Mitchell, P. 'Outdoor Activity Reduces the Prevalence of Myopia in Children', *Ophthalmology* 115 (8), (2008): 1279–85. https://doi.org/10.1016/j.ophtha.2007.12.019.

Rosen, G. 'Changing Attitudes of the Medical Profession to Specialization', *Bulletin of the History of Medicine* 12 (2), (1942): 343–54.

Rosenfeld, P. J.; Brown, D. M.; Heier, J. S.; Boyer, D. S.; Kaiser, P. K.; Chung, C. Y.; Kim, R. Y.; MARINA Study Group. 'Ranibizumab for Neovascular Age-Related Macular Degeneration', *New England Journal of Medicine* 355 (14), (2006): 1419–31. https://doi.org/10.1056/NEJMoa054481.

Royal National Institute for the Blind. 'Information for Employers'. https://www.rnib.org.uk/employers-and-businesses/employing-blind-or-partially-sighted-person. Accessed 22 June 2022.

Rubin, G. S.; Feely, M.; Perera, S.; Ekstrom, K.; Williamson, E. 'The Effect of Font and Line Width on Reading Speed in People with Mild to Moderate Vision Loss', *Ophthalmic and Physiological Optics* 26 (6), (2006): 545–54. https://doi.org/10.1111/j.1475-1313.2006.00409.x.

Rubin, G. S.; Legge, G. E. 'Psychophysics of Reading. VI – The Role of Contrast in Low Vision', *Vision Research* 29 (1), (1989): 79–91. https://doi.org/10.1016/0042-6989(89)90175-2.

Rubin, G. S.; Turano, K. 'Low Vision Reading with Sequential Word Presentation', *Vision Research* 34 (13), (1994): 1723–33. https://doi.org/10.1016/0042-6989(94)90129-5.

Ruiz-Comellas, A.; Valmaña, G. S.; Catalina, Q. M.; Baena, I. G.; Peña, J. M.; Poch, P. R.; Carrera, A. S. et al. 'Effects of Physical Activity Interventions in the Elderly with Anxiety, Depression, and Low Social Support: A Clinical Multicentre Randomised Trial', *Healthcare* 10 (11), (2022): 2203. https://doi.org/10.3390/healthcare10112203.

Sarwar, H.; Modi, N. 'Sir Harold Ridley: Innovator of Cataract Surgery', *Journal of Perioperative Practice* 24 (9), (2014): 210–12. https://doi.org/10.1177/175045891402400905.

Schémann, J. F.; Bakayoko, S.; Coulibaly, S. 'Traditional Couching Is Not an Effective Alternative Procedure for Cataract Surgery in Mali', *Ophthalmic Epidemiology* 7 (4), (2000): 271–83. https://doi.org/10.1076/opep.7.4.271.4174.

Schimansky, S.; Bennetto, L.; Harrison, R. 'Palinopsia', *Practical Neurology* 22 (5), (2022): 392–95. https://doi.org/10.1136/practneurol-2022-003347.

Schmidt-Erfurth, U.; Garcia-Arumi, J.; Gerendas, B. S.; Midena, E.; Sivaprasad, S.; Tadayoni, R.; Wolf, S.; Loewenstein, A. 'Guidelines for the Management of Retinal Vein Occlusion by the European Society of Retina Specialists (EURETINA)', *Ophthalmologica* 242 (3), (2019): 123–62. https://doi.org/10.1159/000502041.

Schuch, F. B.; Stubbs, B. 'The Role of Exercise in Preventing and Treating Depression', *Current Sports Medicine Reports* 18 (8), (2019): 299–304. https://doi.org/10.1249/JSR.0000000000000620.

Seabrook, J. 'What Should a Nine-Thousand-Pound Electric Vehicle Sound Like?'. *The New Yorker*, 8 August 2022.

Sengupta, M. '"Making Art Accessible": India's First Braille Graffiti at Jadaypur University', *Live Wire*, 19 March 2020. https://livewire.thewire.in/campus/making-art-accessible-indias-first-braille-graffiti-at-jadavpur-university. Accessed 16 October 2023.

Shaw, A.; Gold, D.; Wolffe, K. 'Employment-Related Experiences of Youths Who Are Visually Impaired: How Are These Youths Faring?', *Journal of Visual Impairment & Blindness* 101 (1), (2007): 7–21. https://doi.org/10.1177/0145482X0710100103.

Shim, S. H.; Kim, G.; Lee, D. R.; Lee, J. E.; Kwon, H. J.; Song, W. K. 'Survival of Transplanted Human Embryonic Stem Cell-Derived Retinal Pigment Epithelial Cells in a Human Recipient for 22 Months', *JAMA Ophthalmology* 135 (3), (2017): 287–89. https://doi.org/10.1001/jamaophthalmol.2016.5824.

Silverstein, S.; Wang, Y.; Roche, M. 'Base Rates, Blindness, and Schizophrenia', *Frontiers in Psychology* 4 (2013). https://www.frontiersin.org/articles/10.3389/fpsyg.2013.00157/full.

Slade, J.; Edwards, R. 'My Voice 2015: The Views and Experiences of Blind and Partially Sighted People in the UK'. Royal National Institute for Blind People, 2015. https://www.rnib.org.uk/professionals/health-social-care-education-professionals/knowledge-and-research-hub/reports-and-insight/my-voice/.

Sleath, B.; Blalock, S. J.; Stone, J. L.; Skinner, A. C.; Covert, D.; Muir, K.; Robin, A. L. 'Validation of a Short Version of the Glaucoma Medication Self-Efficacy Questionnaire', *British Journal of Ophthalmology* 96 (2), (2012): 258–62. https://doi.org/10.1136/bjo.2010.199851.

Smith, D. J.; Nicholl, B. I.; Cullen, B.; Martin, D.; Ul-Haq, Z.; Evans, J.; Gill, J. M. R. et al. 'Prevalence and Characteristics of Probable Major Depression and Bipolar Disorder within UK

Biobank: Cross-Sectional Study of 172,751 Participants', *PLoS One* 8 (11), (2013): e75362. https://doi.org/10.1371/journal.pone.0075362.

Smith, L.; Shin, J. I.; Barnett, Y.; Allen, P. M.; Lindsay, R.; Pizzol, D.; Jacob, L. et al. 'Association of Objective Visual Impairment with Suicidal Ideation and Suicide Attempts among Adults Aged ≥50 Years in Low/Middle-Income Countries', *British Journal of Ophthalmology* 106 (11), (2022): 1610–16. https://doi.org/10.1136/bjophthalmol-2021-318864.

Sorokowska, A. 'Olfactory Performance in a Large Sample of Early-Blind and Late-Blind Individuals', *Chemical Senses* 41 (8), (2016): 703–9. https://doi.org/10.1093/chemse/bjw081.

Sorokowska, A.; Sorokowski, P.; Karwowski, M.; Larsson, M.; Hummel, T. 'Olfactory Perception and Blindness: A Systematic Review and Meta-Analysis', *Psychological Research* 83 (8), (2019): 1595–611. https://doi.org/10.1007/s00426-018-1035-2.

Sorsby, A. 'On the Nature of Milton's Blindness', *British Journal of Ophthalmology* 14 (7), (1930): 339–54. https://doi.org/10.1136/bjo.14.7.339.

Spiers, N.; Qassem, T.; Bebbington, P.; McManus, S.; King, M.; Jenkins, R.; Meltzer, H.; Brugha, T. S. 'Prevalence and Treatment of Common Mental Disorders in the English National Population, 1993–2007', *British Journal of Psychiatry* 209 (2), (2016): 150–56. https://doi.org/10.1192/bjp.bp.115.174979.

Spratt, A.; Ogunbowale, L.; Khawaja, A.; Franks, W. 'Drops and Falls', *Age and Ageing* 35 (6), (2006): 646. https://doi.org/10.1093/ageing/afl113.

Stalvey, M. L. S. 'Love Is Not Blind: Eugenics, Blindness, and Marriage in the United States, 1840–1940', *ProQuest*, 2014. https://search.proquest.com/docview/1615376062?pq-origsite=primo. Accessed 10 January 2023.

Stoerig, P.; Cowey, A. 'Blindsight', *Current Biology* 17 (19), (2007): R822–24. https://doi.org/10.1016/j.cub.2007.07.016.

Strawbridge, W. J.; Wallhagen, M. I.; Shema, S. J. 'Impact of Spouse Vision Impairment on Partner Health and Well-Being: A Longitudinal Analysis of Couples', *Journals of Gerontology: Series B* 62 (5), (2007): S315–22. https://doi.org/10.1093/geronb/62.5.S315.

Stroffregen, T. A.; Pittenger, J. B. 'Human Echolocation as a Basic Form of Perception and Action', *Ecological Psychology* 7 (3), (1995): 181–216. https://doi.org/10.1207/s15326969eco0703_2.

Tadić, V.; Hundt, G. L.; Keeley, S.; Rahi, J. S.; Vision-Related Quality of Life (VQoL) group. 'Seeing It My Way: Living with Childhood Onset Visual Disability', *Child: Care Health and Development* 41 (2), (2015): 239–48. https://doi.org/10.1111/cch.12158.

Takeuchi, K. 'Pre-Implantation Genetic Testing: Past, Present, Future', *Reproductive Medicine and Biology* 20 (1), (2021): 27–40. https://doi.org/10.1002/rmb2.12352.

Tanna, P.; Strauss, R. W.; Fujinami, K.; Michaelides, M. 'Stargardt Disease: Clinical Features, Molecular Genetics, Animal Models and Therapeutic Options', *British Journal of Ophthalmology* 101 (1), (2017): 25–30. https://doi.org/10.1136/bjophthalmol-2016-308823.

Tarkkanen, A. 'Blindness of Johann Sebastian Bach', *Acta Ophthalmologica* 91 (2), (2013): 191–92. https://doi.org/10.1111/j.1755-3768.2011.02366.x.

The Guide Horse Foundation. 'The Guide Horse Foundation'. Accessed 14 December 2022. http://www.guide-horse.org.

'The Secret Life of Sue Townsend (Aged 68¾)', 2016. https://www.bbc.co.uk/programmes/b080391j. Accessed 11 May 2022.

'Thomas Rhodes Armitage', *British Medical Journal* 2 (1557), (1890): 1039–40. https://www.ncbi.nlm.nih.gov/pmc/articles/PMC2208378/.

Thomas, P. B. M.; Nesaratnam, N.; Chaudhuri-Vayalambrone, P.; Mollon, J. D. 'Color Vision Deficiency among Doctors: Can We Make Useful Adaptations to the Color Codes Used in the Clinical Environment?', *Journal of Patient Safety* 17 (8), (2021): e1646. https://doi.org/10.1097/PTS.0000000000000611.

Thomson, R. *The Insult*. London: Bloomsbury, 1996.

Tiller, J. W. G. 'Depression and Anxiety', *Medical Journal of Australia* 199 (S6), (2013): S28–31. https://doi.org/10.5694/mja12.10628.

Torre, J. A. D. L.; Vilagut, G.; Ronaldson, A.; Serrano-Blanco, A.; Valderas, J.; Martín, V.; Dregan, A.; Bakolis, I.; Alonso, J. 'Prevalence of Depression in Europe Using Two Different PHQ-8 Scoring Methods', *European Psychiatry* 65 (S1), (2022): S299. https://doi.org/10.1192/j.eurpsy.2022.763.

Townsend, S. *Adrian Mole and the Weapons of Mass Destruction*. London: Penguin, 2004.

Townsend, S. *The Public Confessions of a Middle-Aged Woman (Aged 55¾)*. London: Penguin, 2012.

Transport for London. 'Tube Map Large Print (Black and White)'. 2022. https://content.tfl.gov.uk/bw-large-print-tube-map.pdf.

Trevor-Roper, P. *The World through Blunted Sight*, 3rd ed. London: Souvenir Press, 1997.

Uber. 'Global Citizenship'. https://www.uber.com/gb/en/community. Accessed 6 December 2022.

Under the Same Sun. 'What We Do'. www.underthesamesun.com/content/advocacy-public-awareness. Accessed 7 June 2022.

United Nations. 'Convention on the Rights of Persons with Disabilities'. https://www.un.org/development/desa/disabilities/convention-on-the-rights-of-persons-with-disabilities/convention-on-the-rights-of-persons-with-disabilities-2.html. Accessed 22 June 2022.

van der Aa, H. P. A.; van Rens, G. H. M. B.; Comijs, H. C.; Margrain, T. H.; Gallindo-Garre, F.; Twisk, J. W. R.; van Nispen, R. M. A. 'Stepped Care for Depression and Anxiety in Visually Impaired Older Adults: Multicentre Randomised Controlled Trial', *BMJ* 351, (2015): h6127. https://doi.org/10.1136/bmj.h6127.

van der Ham, A. J.; van der Aa, H. P. A.; Verstraten, P.; van Rens, G. H. M. B.; van Nispen, R. M. A. 'Experiences with Traumatic Events, Consequences and Care among People with Visual Impairment and Post-Traumatic Stress Disorder: A Qualitative Study from the Netherlands', *BMJ Open* 11 (2), (2021): e041469. https://doi.org/10.1136/bmjopen-2020-041469.

van der Ham, A. J.; van der Aa, H. P.; Brunes, A.; Heir, T.; de Vries, R.; van Rens, G. H.; van Nispen, R. M. 'The Development of Posttraumatic Stress Disorder in Individuals with Visual Impairment: A Systematic Search and Review', *Ophthalmic and Physiological Optics* 41 (2), (2021): 331–41. https://doi.org/10.1111/opo.12784.

Velichkovsky, B. M.; Zinchenko, V. P. 'New Perspectives on Cognitive Psychology', *Studies in Logic and the Foundations of Mathematics*, 104, (1982): 571–82. https://doi.org/10.1016/S0049-237X(09)70220-4.

Venkatesh, R.; van Landingham, S. W.; Khodifad, A. M.; Haripriya, A.; Thiel, C. L.; Ramulu, P.; Robin, A. L. 'Carbon Footprint and Cost–Effectiveness of Cataract Surgery', *Current Opinion in Ophthalmology* 27 (1), (2016): 82–88. https://doi.org/10.1097/ICU.0000000000000228.

'View from the Boundary – Peter White', *Test Match Special*, 27 August 2022. https://www.bbc.co.uk/programmes/p0cwtlbt.

Voisin, A.; Pénaguin, A.; Gaillard, A.; Leveziel, N. 'Stem Cell Therapy in Retinal Diseases', *Neural Regeneration Research* 18 (7), (2023): 1478–85. https://doi.org/10.4103/1673-5374.361537.

Voss, P.; Lassonde, M.; Gougoux, F.; Fortin, M.; Guillemot, J.-P.; Lepore, F. 'Early- and Late-Onset Blind Individuals Show Supra-Normal Auditory Abilities in Far-Space', *Current Biology* 14 (19), (2004): 1734–38. https://doi.org/10.1016/j.cub.2004.09.051.

Walker, R.; Bryan, L.; Harvey, H.; Riazi, A.; Anderson, S. J. 'The Value of Tablets as Reading Aids for Individuals with Central Visual Field Loss: An Evaluation of Eccentric Reading with Static and Scrolling Text', *Ophthalmic Physiological Optics* 36 (4), (2016): 459–64. https://doi.org/10.1111/opo.12296.

Wan, C. Y.; Wood, A. G.; Reutens, D. C.; Wilson, S. J. 'Early but Not Late-Blindness Leads to Enhanced Auditory Perception', *Neuropsychologia* 48 (1), (2010): 344–48. https://doi.org/10.1016/j.neuropsychologia.2009.08.016.

WeCapable. 'Disability in Japan: Laws, Rights, Discrimination and Stigma'. https://wecapable.com/disability-in-japan-laws-rights-discrimination-and-stigma. Accessed 22 June 2022.

Weiskrantz, L.; Warrington, E. K.; Sanders, M. D.; Marshall, J. 'Visual Capacity in the Hemianopic Field Following a Restricted Occipital Ablation', *Brain* 97 (1), (1974): 709–28. https://doi.org/10.1093/brain/97.1.709.

White, P. *See It My Way*. London: Little, Brown and Company, 1999.

World Health Organization. 'ICD-11: International Classification of Diseases' (11th Revision), 2019. https://icd.who.int/en.

Wynick, S.; Hobson, R. P.; Jones, R. B. 'Psychogenic Disorders of Vision in Childhood ("Visual Conversion Reactions"): Perspectives from Adolescence: A Research Note', *Journal of Child Psychology and Psychiatry* 38 (3), (1997): 375–79. https://doi.org/10.1111/j.1469-7610.1997.tb01521.x.

'Xalatan Prices, Coupons and Patient Assistance Programs', Drugs.com. Accessed 31 January 2023. https://www.drugs.com/price-guide/xalatan.

Yang, Y.; Ton, C.; Omar, A.; Szedenko, V.; Tran, V. H.; Aftab, A. 'Performance Analysis of LIDAR Assist Spatial Sensing for the Visually Impaired', *Proceedings* 1 (8), (2017): 774. https://doi.org/10.3390/proceedings1080774.

Zhou, Z.; Chen, T.; Wang, M.; Jin, L.; Zhao, Y.; Chen, S.; Wang, C. et al. 'Pilot Study of a Novel Classroom Designed to Prevent Myopia by Increasing Children's Exposure to Outdoor Light', *PLoS One* 12 (7), (2017): e0181772. https://doi.org/10.1371/journal.pone.0181772.

Index

optometrists, 8, 11, 75, 77, 119, 123, 126
orthoptists, 12

Pacino, Al, 25
Palinopsia, 74
Papalia, Carmen, 100–101, 126
parenting with vision impairment, 46–48, 83
perfume, 26, 51–52
piano playing, 29, 36, 59, 120
post-traumatic stress disorder (PTSD), 87
posterior cortical atrophy, 75
pregnancy, 51
prisms, 68, 70–71, 79
prison, 28, 92–93, 95–96
prison officers, 41
prosopagnosia (face blindness), 73

rapid serial visual presentation (RSVP), 60
Read-Right (computer programme), 79
reasonable adjustments (workplaces), 39, 41
retinal vein occlusion, 112, 115
retinitis pigmentosa, 51, 81, 90, 117
retinopathy of prematurity (ROP), 27
Richie, Lionel, 20
Royal National Institute for Blind People, 2, 36, 42, 61, 88
Royal Normal College and Academy for the Blind, 36, 37, 42

Sacks, Oliver, xiii
Scent of a Woman (film), 25–26
schizophrenia, 74, 91–92
sculpture, 20–23
Seeing AI, 123–125
Shakespeare, Tom, xiii
sign language, 57
simulating vision impairment, 13, 19, 20, 31
smell, sense of, 22, 51–53

Snellen chart, 3–5
spatial neglect, 69–70, 71
Stargardt disease, 1, 117, 118
stem cell therapy, 115–116
Stevens-Johnson syndrome, 53
suicidal ideation, 87–88
suicide, 26, 88
syphilis, 29, 83, 95

tactile
    acuity, 55, 57
    avoidance, 29
    drawings, 22–24
    markings on bank notes, 28
    teaching tools, 39
    writing, 104, *see also* braille
Tagliaferri, Felice, 21–22
taste, sense of, 22, 53
taxis, 40, 46, 99, 100, 106
teachers, 6, 13, 20, 37, 38, 40, 95
    art teachers, 20, 25
    careers teachers, 17, 36
    teachers for vision impairment, 1, 11, 12, 22, 59
Thomas, Peter, 42
Thomson, Rupert, 69
Tinder, 106
Tiresias (font), 61
Tiresias (historical character), 62
'Touch to See' books, 22
touch, sense of, 29, 53, 55, 56, 57, 67, 70, 122
Touching the Rock (book), 47, 63
Townsend, Sue, 30–31, 144
travelling, 103–106
Trevor-Roper, Patrick, 17
Tsujii, Nobuyuki, 29
tunnel vision, 3, 8, 60

Uber, 100
United Nations Convention on the Rights of Persons with Disabilities, 39

Valsalva manoeuvre, 83–84
Vanga, Baba, 63
visual acuity, 3–6, 42, 55, 56, 68, 74–75, 109, 118, 125

visual cortex, 52, 55–56, 67, 72–73
visual field, 3, 6–8, 20, 28, 42, 51, 67–72, 89, 118
von Trier, Lars, 26
Vonnegut, Kurt, 7

Wales House, 47
Walker, Robin, 60
white canes, 8, 31, 43, 51, 63, 100–102, 106
White, Peter, 35, 36, 37, 100
Wonder, Stevie, 27–29

workplaces
    vision impairment caused by, 43–46
    visual standards for, 41–42
    working with vision impairment, 39–41
World Health Organization, 5, 6, 28, 42

'Yes But' game, 85

Zatōichi, 25, 63

Printed in the USA
CPSIA information can be obtained
at www.ICGtesting.com
CBHW052327130924
13897CB00011B/21